Foundations for 21st-Century Healh and Social Care

This comprehensive text introduces health and social care theory and practice for students studying at foundation degree level, including those on nursing associate and assistant practitioner pathways.

Keeping themes of professionalism and patient-centred care at its core, this text equips readers to deliver effective, safe and responsive care in a wide range of settings. It anticipates future directions for practice and provides readers with skills they will need throughout their careers. Divided into four parts, it explores the foundations of academic study, becoming and being a professional, working with patients and service users and improving services and improving health.

Clearly presented and reader-friendly, this textbook is an essential companion for all health and social care students.

Dr Lisa Arai is a social and public health scientist with 25 years' research and teaching experience. Her research interests are in the health of children and young people. She is based at Solent University and the University of Northampton in the United Kingdom. Lisa has published widely and is a Fellow of the Royal Society for Public Health.

Foundations for 21st-Century Health and Social Care

Theory and Practice for Nursing Associates, Assistant Practitioners, Support Workers and Beyond

Edited by Lisa Arai

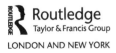

Routledge
Taylor & Francis Group

LONDON AND NEW YORK

Cover image: Tamsin Arai Drake

First published 2024
by Routledge
4 Park Square, Milton Park, Abingdon, Oxon OX14 4RN

and by Routledge
605 Third Avenue, New York, NY 10158

Routledge is an imprint of the Taylor & Francis Group, an informa business

British Library Cataloguing-in-Publication Data
A catalogue record for this book is available from the British Library

Library of Congress Cataloging-in-Publication Data
Names: Arai, Lisa, editor.
Title: Foundations for 21st-Century Health and Social Care
Theory and Practice for Nursing Associates, Assistant Practitioners,
Support Workers and Beyond / edited by Lisa Arai.
Other titles: Foundations for twenty-first century health and social care
Description: Abingdon, Oxon ; New York, NY : Routledge, 2024. |
Includes bibliographical references and index.
Identifiers: LCCN 2023010806 | ISBN 9781032056111 (hardback) |
ISBN 9781032056005 (paperback) | ISBN 9781003198338 (ebook)
Subjects: LCSH: Nursing–Study and teaching–Great Britain. |
Medical care–Great Britain. | Social services–Great Britain.
Classification: LCC RT81.G7 F678 2024 |
DDC 610.73–dc23/eng/20230606
LC record available at https://lccn.loc.gov/2023010806

ISBN: 978-1-032-05611-1 (hbk)
ISBN: 978-1-032-05600-5 (pbk)
ISBN: 978-1-003-19833-8 (ebk)

DOI: 10.4324/9781003198338

Typeset in Sabon
by Newgen Publishing UK

Contents

Contributor biographies

Gemma Burley is based at Solent University in the United Kingdom. She is the course lead for the health and social care foundation degree and is a registered adult nurse. She leads on anatomy and physiology modules well as those focused on supervision and assessment in practice.

Dr Teresa Corbett is based at Solent University in the United Kingdom. Teresa is a chartered psychologist specialising in health psychology. To date, her work has largely focused on the development of interventions promoting quality of life of patients living with complex long-term conditions. This has led to an interest in person-centred care and to exploring the challenges to implementing this approach in practice.

Ann Gorecki is a senior lecturer for the foundation degree in health and social care at Solent University in the United Kingdom. She was a registered adult nurse before moving into teaching in further education and, for the last seven years, has taught in higher education on early years and health and social care courses.

Dr Kieron Hatton is a lecturer in social work at Solent University in the United Kingdom. He is a registered social worker and Fellow of Advance HE and has been a social work academic for 30 years. His areas of research include UK and international social work, social pedagogy, youth work and community development. Kieron has a particular interest in ensuring service users have a 'voice' and are able to exercise control over the services they use.

Margaret Johanson has worked at Solent University in the United Kingdom for almost 30 years as a buyer for ICT equipment. After years of pain, she was diagnosed with fibromyalgia. As a member of Solent University's Service User Group, she shares her experiences of this long-term health condition so that healthcare professional students have an insight of the impact this disease can have on physical and mental health.

Mandy Lyons is based at Solent University in the United Kingdom and is a registered nurse and educator who has championed the development of healthcare assistants while working within the NHS and higher education. She has led nursing associate education since the original pilot programme was launched by Health Education England and strives to widen participation in higher education to support professional development.

Dr Lindsay Welch is based at the Faculty of Environmental and Life Sciences at the University of Southampton in the United Kingdom. She is a lecturer in adult nursing and a researcher in the field of long-term conditions. Lindsay is a specialist respiratory nurse and has worked for over 20 years in clinical practice before she was appointed to her current academic role.

Figures

Tables

1 Introduction

Lisa Arai

Welcome and aim of this book

Welcome to this book, entitled *Foundations for 21st-Century Health and Social Care: Theory and Practice for Nursing Associates, Assistant Practitioners, Support Workers and Beyond*. This book's aim is to explore the main areas of health and social care (H&SC) theory and practice so that current and future practitioners are equipped to deliver effective, safe and responsive care in a diverse range of settings in 21st-century United Kingdom (UK).

To reach this aim, this book will examine a range of practical and theoretical areas relevant for learners. It covers diverse areas of H&SC practice, from clinical aspects to the more sociological, and it has a central focus on developing professionalism and the skills needed to be a person-centred practitioner. Other areas explored here include essential study skills, working of the human body and public health and health promotion.

The audience for this book

While the primary audience for this textbook are students taking a H&SC foundation degree[1]—or future learners on such programmes—anyone with an interest in this subject (either practical or theoretical) is likely to find this book useful. Many H&SC programmes in the UK don't have a practice element; students on these programmes focus solely on theoretical aspects of H&SC. Such students are invited to explore this book and are likely to be particularly interested in the more theoretical chapters.

This book is relevant for a UK-based (primarily English) audience but draws on international research and refers to H&SC practice in other nations. Some chapters (like the one focused on study skills or that on the 'nuts and bolts' of the human body) are relevant for all learners regardless of which country they reside in.

Background to the book

Most chapter authors are based at Solent University in Southampton, UK, or have strong links with the university. Solent-based authors teach two main groups of student practitioners on its highly regarded[2] H&SC foundation degree programme: trainee nursing associates (TNAs) and healthcare assistant practitioners (HCAPs). We also teach nursing students and learners on other practice-oriented programmes (such as social work) on an *ad hoc* basis. TNAs and HCAPs must be in practice to be eligible to join the programme, and TNAs must complete placements in addition to working in their

DOI: 10.4324/9781003198338-1

primary workplace. Most students are apprentices, and all are released from the workplace for a day in a week to study on the programme.

Our students work in a variety of clinical settings such as paediatrics, maternity, primary care, older people's care and in the community. All these settings are heavily regulated by various professional, statutory and regulatory bodies (PSRBs) such as the Nursing and Midwifery Council (NMC)[3] and the Health and Care Professions Council (HCPC). Other stakeholders include Health Education England, who were the first PSRB to assume responsibility for nursing associates.

As learners and practitioners (most with many years' clinical practice experience and extensive practice-related knowledge), our students are especially hard-working. Most are female and mature and have responsibilities for children and elderly parents; as such, they juggle many roles. Only a small percentage of the students we've taught at Solent have prior experience of higher education, and some have not interacted with the education system since completion of General Certificate of Secondary Education or 'O' level qualifications.

These characteristics of our student body present challenges for learners and academic staff alike. Students often struggle with foundational academic skills, such as academic writing or referencing, or lack confidence in their ability to learn. Students also often worry about meeting deadlines when they are in practice most of the week (although all have protected learning time). Academic staff teaching these learners sometimes don't know how best to support them and might be insufficiently aware of practice-related issues affecting academic performance.

This book was borne out of our many years' experience of teaching these types of practitioner students. We intended to develop a textbook that could reflect the structure and content of our NMC-validated programme, that could be a hands-on learning resource and that could also help our students understand *all* aspects of being a student—especially the foundational skills mentioned above—rather than just programme-related practice and theory. However, while this book has a broad scope and is comprehensive, it does not (and cannot) cover everything needed for learners on these and similar programmes. We do not cover clinical skills, for example. You are advised to consult authoritative and well-regarded texts, such as that produced by The Royal Marsden NHS Foundation Trust (2020).

We also wanted to reach a wider audience with an interest in H&SC. This is an important area of research, practice and professional activity. It's a broad discipline that includes students studying subjects such as nursing and allied health health studies, public health and social work. Students may be either work-based (apprentices) or, as noted earlier, learning on theory-only programmes (although many students even on non–practice-oriented H&SC programmes have at least one placement).

Health and social care workforce in the UK

The Solent-based authors and their colleagues in other institutions are helping train the H&SC workforce of the future. What does this workforce look like? What are the challenges they face in their everyday practice with patients and service users?

Health and social care workforce

In relation to the first question, the H&SC workforce in the UK has grown and become increasingly diverse over time. Many healthcare roles and associate roles (in particular) have expanded over the last few years. H&SC workers can be found in diverse, clinical areas in hospitals, primary care, the community, older people's residential homes, prisons and hospices. HCAPs can often be found in laboratories, specialist therapy areas and mental health settings. All these practitioners perform challenging, vital and, sometimes, overlooked (but enormously rewarding) work. Practitioners at bands 2–4[4] deliver most of the care needed for the efficient running of the National Health Service (NHS). Without them, the NHS and other care organisations would likely collapse.

Career progression has not always been straightforward for this group of workers. In the recent past, healthcare assistants have had little opportunity to advance beyond their role (despite developing expertise over many years' clinical practice). The nursing associate role was developed to offer band 2 workers a way to develop and upgrade their skills and engage in more demanding clinical practice (Glasper 2017). This relatively new addition to the healthcare family (TNAs began their training in England in 2016) also frees up nurses to work with patients with more complex needs.

In addition to developing clearer career progression pathways for H&SC practitioners, there has been a national drive to boost the number of H&SC workers. Issues around poor staffing were especially acute during the COVID-19 pandemic; indeed, one of the drivers for the lockdown was the fear that the NHS would be overwhelmed by the sheer number of people needing medical facilities. Also, the experience of living through a pandemic and seeing loved ones being treated has led to increasing interest in nursing and other areas of care (Kale 2020). This is to be welcomed: care work is rewarding and important, and there is a great need for compassionate and committed H&SC professionals. Meeting the educational, practice and other needs of these workers is paramount.

Challenges faced by health and social care workers

The challenges that H&SC workers face are growing and it's imperative that educators help equip their students with the skills to meet these. The chief challenge is an increasing number of older patients with multiple morbidities whose care typically involves a diverse range of practitioners. Because of the scope and nature of these patients' conditions and their growing numbers, it's important not only to 'grow' the practitioner workforce to ensure that there are enough *"hands on deck"* to care for this group but also to train them to address the specific clinical, social and psychological needs of this population. The numbers are stark: the population of the UK aged over 65 years was approximately 12 million in 2019 (19% of the UK population). By 2043, this group will increase to 24% of the population, and 13% of people will be aged 75 years and older (an increase from 8% in 2018) (House of Commons Library 2021).

Other challenges H&SC practitioners must navigate include working in often high-pressured clinical settings where multiple demands are made of their time and energy and where patient expectations are high (Duffy 2018). Yet, despite these growing expectations, practitioners increasingly find themselves working in (relatively speaking) low-resource settings. The issue of NHS funding is a fraught one (and it will not be considered here). There are some commentators who point to increased funding for the NHS in recent years, while others highlight the lower proportion of the UK's gross domestic product (GDP) spent on healthcare compared with other developed Western nations (see Savage 2022 for discussion of spending on the NHS and comparisons with other countries).

Whatever the issues around funding of the NHS, H&SC professionals' accounts of working practices reported in research and policy outputs often highlight the impact of a lack of resources, low staff numbers and poor working conditions on staff morale. The Royal College of Nursing (RCN) annual survey of members' employment experiences, for example, often reports generally negative experiences including high workload and harassment by colleagues and patients. Of over 9,000 responses from RCN members in 2021, 74.1% reported regularly working beyond their contracted hours at least once a week, with 17.4% doing so in every shift or working day. Nearly 67% of respondents said that they felt under too much pressure at work and 61.5% said they're too busy to provide the level of care they would like to (Royal College of Nursing 2021).

The situation is not likely to change soon for H&SC workers. At the time of writing, the UK (and most other countries) were experiencing cost-of-living and energy crises partly brought about by the war in Ukraine, and the UK government debt had grown to £2,436.7 billion by June 2022, equivalent to 101.9% of GDP (Office for National Statistics 2022). Nurses were planning a strike for the first time in their history. Given these considerable challenges, it is especially important that H&SC practitioners are supported by clinical and academic educators to become the most efficient, knowledge-able, professional and collegiate professionals they can be.

Overview of chapters and engaging with this book

Overview of chapters

There are four parts to this book: 'The foundations of academic study', 'Becoming and being a professional', 'Patients and service users: At the heart of H&SC' and 'Improving services, improving health'. After this introductory chapter, there are 12 chapters.

Part 1: The foundations of academic study

In chapter 2, Lisa Arai (who has been teaching since 2004) examines the essential study skills. These are foundational skills that, if not developed by students early on in their academic career, can compromise educational achievement. These are also skills that need to be continually revisited and developed, especially as learners transition from one year (and level) to the next. Arai categorises academic skills into 'preparing', 'researching' and 'writing up'. She considers a range of skills falling into each of these three areas.

Chapter 3 focuses on students' use of research evidence and designing small-scale research projects. Many foundation degree students are not *directly* involved in research. However, students must draw on research evidence to support observations made in academic assignments. To do this effectively requires a basic understanding of how research evidence is generated. Practitioners are also required to be 'evidence-based' in their practice (this central concept in H&SC practice is examined in this chapter). Lisa Arai, who was a researcher before she became a lecturer, examines what the terms 'research' and 'research evidence' mean and explores the use of research evidence in academic study.

Part 2: Becoming and being a professional

The second part of the book focuses on the transition to professional status and the experience of being a professional.

In chapter 4, Ann Gorecki, an experienced educator with an adult nursing background, discusses the policy and legislative backdrop to H&SC practice in the UK. As noted above, H&SC professionals are heavily regulated by PSRBs and must abide by a diverse array of regulations. They are also subject to workplace policies and national legislation. Gorecki discusses the relevance of policy and legislation to practitioners and provides a brief history of key legislation from 1946 to the present day. She also assesses future legislative developments and considers their potential impact on current services.

Mandy Lyons, a NMC registrant, trainer and educator with many years' clinical experience, and Lisa Arai examine key aspects of becoming an H&SC professional in chapter 5. These are embedded in the NMC and other codes and include the requirement for practitioners to be accountable, to practise safe care and to be mindful of their safeguarding and whistleblowing responsibilities. This chapter also considers the process of transitioning from a less to a more regulated role and registration for an NMC PIN.[5] This transition can bring added responsibilities and strains for new registrants, and there is a period of preceptorship for at least a year after transition. While this chapter focuses especially at current or future practitioners, readers not currently in practice or who are not planning to work in an H&SC setting, will benefit from learning about these aspects of professional practice.

H&SC practice inevitably means working closely with others, supervising and mentoring colleagues. These aspects of practice are examined in chapter 6 by Gemma Burley (an academic and NMC registrant with a sexual health nursing background) and Lisa Arai. Burley and Arai explore theories of how people learn, consider H&SC educational roles and discuss different coaching approaches. These authors observe that, while working with others can be challenging, it is ultimately rewarding; there is much to learn from closely working with others, and colleagues are a source of support.

Part 3: Patients and service users: At the heart of health and social care

The five chapters (chapters 7–11) in this part of the book are focused on diverse aspects of clinical, social and emotional care of patients and service users.

A strong, theoretical underpinning knowledge of anatomy and physiology (A&P) is necessary to ensure that H&SC professionals and learners can provide effective care for patients. This includes a comprehensive awareness of the key concepts of A&P in a healthy system and an understanding of the effects of disease and illness on the human body. As writers of chapter 7, Gemma Burley and Mandy Lyons observe, it is impossible to cover A&P in detail within this chapter. This chapter aims to introduce you to key concepts of A&P and provide basic knowledge in preparation for study.

Lindsay Welch, an NMC registrant, lecturer and adult nurse with a special interest in respiratory conditions, discusses long-term conditions (LTCs) and multi morbidity in chapter 8. Welch's chapter introduces the concept of LTCs, discusses why it is important to study LTCs and considers the importance of understanding who is affected by LTCs. She also considers the broader social needs of those with LTCs and the role of the individual in their own care ('self-care' or 'self-management'). Considering the challenges that H&SC professionals face outlined above, this is an increasingly important area of practice.

Chapter 9 focuses on person-centred care (PCC). This paramount concept is explored by Teresa Corbett, a lecturer and researcher at Solent University with a psychology background. PCC recognises and promotes the autonomy of the individual and ensures that 'what matters' to patients is central to their care. Corbett discusses the history and philosophy of PCC and considers potential challenges to its implementation. Whatever the practical challenges of PCC, all professional H&SC bodies and organisations expect it of their members and employees. It is, in many respects, a foundational care concept. Without it, care—even where clinically competent and effective—can lack compassion and compromise the dignity of patients and service users.

Most social work and H&SC students will encounter service users while studying as well as in practice, so it's imperative that they listen to, and engage with, this group. In chapter 10, Kieron Hatton, a social work practitioner and lecturer based at Solent University, and Margaret Walsh, a member of Solent University's Service Users' Group and a person with an LTC, examine the role of service user perspectives in H&SC services and in the training of H&SC professionals. Kieron and Margaret are passionate about care workers hearing, and acting on, service users' accounts of their lives, their conditions and their emotional and physical health needs. Kieron and Margaret explore the history of service user engagement and draw on their own professional and personal experiences in the chapter. Margaret's painful condition was not diagnosed for a long time. As she says: 'It took many years for me to get a diagnosis as my doctor repeatedly told me I was imagining everything which was very demoralising and, in fact, made my symptoms worse'. Kieron utilises insights from training social work students to make the point that people's creativity and imagination can be drawn on to provide unique and insightful educational experiences which have the potential to transform delivery of care.

In chapter 11, Gemma Burley and Lisa Arai explore ethics and ethical dilemmas in H&SC. These authors define 'ethics' and discuss central principles such as autonomy, informed consent and dignity. These principles are especially salient given several high-profile breaches of clinical care contributing to the deaths of patients, such as the Mid Staffordshire ('Mid Staffs') NHS Foundation Trust scandal. The inquiries that were held following such scandals often highlighted the lack of compassion that patients experienced and the harmful practices they were exposed to. Ethical theories are discussed in this chapter, and an ethical framework developed specifically for healthcare settings is examined. Burley and Arai observe that H&SC workers frequently encounter ethical challenges in their everyday practice, that it's rarely easy to resolve ethical dilemmas and, often, there is no one 'right' way to do so. However, good ethical practice is an ongoing requirement of all care providers, especially as H&SC professionals encounter individuals at their most vulnerable, when they are in pain or emotionally distressed.

Part 4: Improving services, improving health

The final part of the book contains two chapters. Lisa Arai, a non-practitioner with a public health research background, defines and explores public health and health promotion in chapter 12. Contemporary public health practice is also examined, and the historical roots of public health, which lie in the 19th century and the first Public Health Act (1848), are discussed. Public health practice relies on the collection and analysis of reliable data to identify threats to health and well-being. Arai considers selected, key concepts relating to health promotion and discusses H&SC practitioners' role in health promotion. This is usually stipulated in the various codes and standards governing their registration and employment.

Importantly, unlike traditional medicine, public health's orientation is preventative rather than curative. Given this, public health recognises the many wider and societal-level factors affecting health and well-being and adopts a 'bird's eye' perspective on health rather than a 'micro', clinical one.

Chapter 13, the final chapter, focuses on service improvement in H&SC settings. Lisa Arai draws on her experience of leading a service improvement module at Solent University to examine this area of activity. She describes selected projects that students have worked on over the years and explores some of the many tools and frameworks to guide would-be service improvers. Chapter 13 focuses on the completion of brief, small-scale and low-cost (or no-cost) projects, ones aimed at reducing waste, increasing efficiency and streamlining aspects of service provision. Importantly, service and quality improvement activities take place against a backdrop of significant challenges to the H&SC services such as those arising from the consequences of an ageing society. These and other 'drivers' of service improvement are examined.

How to engage with this book

All chapters include learning activities and additional resources related to the content of the chapter. To get the most out of this book, please engage with these fully. It's a good idea to have a pen and paper handy when completing activities, as you may be asked to write something. There is no 'right' or 'wrong' answer to the activities. These activities do not aim to 'test' knowledge but to ask you to think about a concept or explore an issue more deeply. You will need access to the Internet to engage with some activities and will be asked to watch videos, so you will need to be able to hear these.

As is the case with most textbooks, you can 'dip into' chapters; there is no need to read chapters in order, although there is some cross-referencing between chapters.

We hope you enjoy this book and that it helps prepare you for H&SC practice and study.

Notes

1 In England, Northern Ireland and Wales, a foundation degree involves studying at levels 4 and 5 (typically, the first 2 years of undergraduate study) (QAA 2014). (See www.qaa.ac.uk/docs/qaa/quality-code/qualifications-frameworks.pdf for more information.) Scotland has a different educational system.
2 The National Student Survey collects the views of final-year undergraduate students in every university in the UK. Solent health and social care students' satisfaction score for 2021 was over 98%.
3 The Nursing and Midwifery Council (NMC) is the professional regulator for nurses and midwives in the UK, and nursing associates in England. (See www.nmc.org.uk/about-us/our-role/ for more information.) All nurses, midwives and nursing associates must be registered with the NMC before they can practise.
4 This refers to the NHS banding structure. (See www.healthcareers.nhs.uk/working-health/working-nhs/nhs-pay-and-benefits/agenda-change-pay-rates/agenda-change-pay-rates for more information.)
5 An NMC PIN is a code given to nurses, nursing associates and midwives so that they can join the NMC register and practise in the UK. (See www.nmc.org.uk/registration/joining-the-register/ for more information.)

References

DUFFY, B., 2018. *Public expectations of the NHS* [viewed 6 January 2023]. Available from: www.kingsfund.org.uk/blog/2018/02/public-expectations-nhs#comments-top

GLASPER, A., 2017. Nurse education and the development of the nursing associate role. *British journal of nursing*, 26(1), 56-57. https://doi.org/10.12968/bjon.2017.26.1.56

HOUSE OF COMMONS LIBRARY, 2021. *Housing an ageing population: A reading list* (briefing paper, number 09239) [viewed 6 January 2023]. Available from: https://researchbriefings.files.parliament.uk/documents/CBP-9239/CBP-9239.pdf

KALE, S., 2020. *In good health: Meet the people who have quit their jobs to join the NHS. The Guardian*, 31st August [viewed 6 January 2023]. Available from: www.theguardian.com/money/2020/aug/31/in-good-health-meet-the-people-who-have-quit-their-jobs-to-join-the-nhs

OFFICE FOR NATIONAL STATISTICS, 2022. *UK government debt and deficit: June 2022: Quarterly estimates of UK government debt and deficit* [viewed 6 January 2023]. Available from: www.ons.gov.uk/economy/governmentpublicsectorandtaxes/publicspending/bulletins/ukgovernmentdebtanddeficitforeurostatmaast/june2022

QUALITY ASSURANCE AGENCY (QAA), 2014. *UK quality code for higher education: Part A: Setting and maintaining academic standards*. Gloucester, UK: QAA.

ROYAL COLLEGE OF NURSING, 2021. *RCN employment survey 2021*. London: RCN.

ROYAL MARSDEN NHS FOUNDATION TRUST, 2020. *The Royal Marsden Manual Online* (10th ed.) [viewed 6 January 2023]. Available from: www.rmmonline.co.uk/

SAVAGE, M., 2022. *NHS crisis caused by Tory underfunding not Covid, say doctors. The Guardian, 26th June* [viewed 6 January 2023]. Available from: www.theguardian.com/society/2022/jun/26/nhs-crisis-caused-by-tory-underfunding-not-covid-say-doctors

Part 1

The Foundations of Academic Study

2 Essential study skills for health and social care students

Lisa Arai

Box 2.1: Contents

- Introduction
- What are the essential study skills?
- Preparing: Laying the groundwork
- Researching: Finding and thinking
- Writing up: Putting it all together
- Dealing with feedback

Box 2.2: Learning outcomes

By the end of this chapter, you should be able to

- Discuss the essential study skills
- Differentiate assignment types
- Understand the elements of academic writing
- Evaluate different types of resources
- Identify ways to use tutor feedback to improve your work.

Box 2.3: Keywords

- Assignment types
- Academic writing
- Referencing
- Proofreading
- Formative feedback
- Summative feedback

DOI: 10.4324/9781003198338-3

Introduction

Some students enter the first year of undergraduate study after being out of the education system for many years. This is especially true of students who are in practice in the health and social care (H&SC) system. These students tend to be older than those in other disciplines. They may have left school or college as teenagers, after gaining General Certificate of Secondary Education (GCSE) or their equivalent, and may have then started working in an H&SC setting (often combining this with raising a family). After some years in their role, these workers may have been offered the chance to further their career by completing a foundation degree or other qualification.

These students are excited by the prospect of re-engaging with education, and they bring a great deal, in terms of practice knowledge and life experience, to the classroom. However, they often lack confidence in respect of academic skills such as identifying and evaluating scholarly resources and referencing and academic writing. In recognition of this, there has been an increasing focus in further and higher education on equipping students with the skills to perform well in their studies. Most universities in the United Kingdom now employ specialist staff to develop study skills materials and run workshops in activities such as searching electronic databases, avoiding plagiarism and effectively managing time.

In this chapter, the essential study skills for H&SC students will be examined. While the focus is on H&SC learners here, these skills are of relevance to *all* students at *all* levels of study. These are also skills that need to be refreshed regularly. It's not uncommon for a student in their final year of study, for example, to continue to make the same errors in referencing or punctuation they made in their earlier years of study. It means that they've not been corrected, not heeded their tutors' instruction or (more commonly), they've forgotten the advice they've been given and reverted to previous erroneous practice (this is especially the case where there is a significant period between submission of assignments). Before we explore specific study skills, let's first examine, more generally, what these skills are.

What are the essential study skills?

What are the study skills that you—as a student commencing level 4 study or continuing study at level 5 and above—need to know about if you are going to pass your assignments? Or (if you are already familiar with these), to practise and develop further (and to keep developing as you progress through your study programme)?

The essential study skills fall (broadly speaking) in three areas (Figure 2.1).

'Preparing' is about understanding the task you are being asked to undertake, especially in respect of the assignment type. It's also about planning the assignment. 'Researching' is the creative and intellectual phase when you identify and evaluate information for your assignment, make notes and formulate ideas. The final phase, 'Writing up', focuses on the actual writing up of your findings, editing and proofreading.

Attaining deep learning

All teaching staff will be familiar with assignment-focused students. These are students who are not interested in learning more generally, so they don't engage fully with module

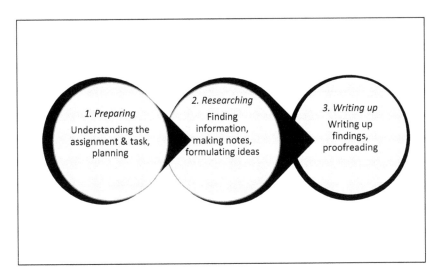

Figure 2.1 Essential study skills
Image credit: Lisa Arai, adapted from: Open Polytechnic (2022)

content or participate in classroom activities and are primarily focused on acquiring the knowledge solely to pass the assignment. Cowen, Maier and Price (2013) discuss H&SC learners of this type by reference to motivation:

> Your degree of motivation for your subject will determine how you study and how much effort you put in. If you are not very motivated, you will more than likely be someone who will memorise enough facts to get you through the coursework and exams; you will be what is called a 'surface learner', take little time to reflect on your learning, have a 'make-do' attitude to your studies and have difficulty managing your commitments (p.9).

These authors observe that such a person is not the ideal student, or the ideal employee and his or her lack of motivation will be evident to academic staff as well as potential employers. Moreover, they note, H&SC practitioner students may attempt to justify this lack of motivation by claiming that, as they are entering a caring profession, all they need is a caring manner. On the contrary, these authors write, patients and employers deserve knowledgeable practitioners.

As for assignment writing, the same 'surface learners' may attempt to bypass the first two stages named above ('preparing' and 'researching') and progress straight to the writing up stage. This is a mistake, one that's usually evident from the quality of the assignment. The key message that this chapter provides to its learners is: Don't rush to write up; take your time when starting the work for your assignment and ensure that you progress through all stages. We will look at each of these in detail now.

Activity 2.1: What helps boost your motivation?

Are you a 'surface' learner? If you are, what might motivate you to become a deeper learner? Make a list of the things that might help boost your motivation.

Preparing: laying the groundwork

Understanding assignment types

The first task in this stage is to understand different assignment types and be able to differentiate them. The assignment brief for the module you are studying will refer to the assignment type. The main assignment types and their features are shown in Panel 2.1.

Panel 2.1: Main assignment types and their features

Assignment type	Features
Essay	• Contains a clear introduction, body and conclusion • Often has an argumentative framework • Ideas 'flow' between connected paragraphs • Doesn't usually have sub-headings • Rarely makes recommendations
Report	• Uses a clear structure with sub-headings • Bulleted lists can be used • Usually makes recommendations • Uses a factual, to-the-point writing style • Often has appendices • Can contain images, figures and tables
Presentation	• Can be done as an individual or a group • Depends on effective oral communication • Aids, such as slides, can be used to 'map out' the presentation or illustrate the points prepared • Audience questions are invited at the end of the presentation
Case study	• In-depth examination of one case (such as a patient or service user) • Discusses all aspects of the case's (medical and social) history • Can be used to illustrate a theory or concept • May generalise from the case to a wider group
Examination (including objective structured clinical examination)	• Learners are tested under timed, exam conditions • Usually completed alone • Students advised to revise or practise before the exam • Objective structured clinical examination is a practical exam where learners demonstrate clinical skills in one or more scenarios

---

Essays

Essays are one of the most common types of assignment. Essays are widely used because, as Cottrell (2019, p.319) says, they help students to '… elaborate, structure and present ideas on a given subject, and to develop generic written communication skills. Writing them can sharpen your thinking as well as improve your writing'. She also notes that, as you progress through your programme, there is an expectation that your essay-writing will improve.

Essays usually use an argumentative framework. Cottrell (2019) observes that these essays usually fall into four main areas (see Panel 2.2).

Panel 2.2: Argumentative frameworks in essays

1. For or against: This is where students are asked to argue whether they agree or disagree with a statement (for example, 'The NHS cannot survive in the 21st-century and new models of healthcare delivery are needed'). This essay requires examination of both sides of an argument and weighing up of the evidence before conclusions are drawn
2. To what extent? This framework asks you to judge about how far something is true ('To what extent have public health programmes to reduce child obesity been effective?')
3. Compare and contrast: The student here is being asked to examine similarities and differences in something ('Compare and contrast pharmacological treatments for childhood asthma')
4. Reflective essay: This is a specific type of essay widely used in H&SC. All practitioners are required to be reflective (the Nursing and Midwifery Standards of Proficiency for Nursing Associates, for example, requires nursing associates to: '…take responsibility for continuous self-reflection, seeking and responding to support and feedback to develop professional knowledge and skills knowledge and skills') (Nursing and Midwifery Council 2018). In a reflective essay, the student draws on their practice experience to demonstrate an aspect of professional development (such as how they developed confidence while caring for a patient, for example, or how they learned to deal with a challenging situation). Importantly, the reflection is undertaken to show learning from a situation and how the practitioner would deal with the situation if encountered again

Adapted from: Cottrell (2019).

The exact format of essays varies by discipline, but all essays contain prose connected by paragraphs. Paragraphs are generally considered the building blocks of essays (McMillan and Weyers 2012) and are used to establish a sense of 'flow'. It's not always easy to do this; many students find that, when they first start writing essays, their ideas 'jump around' and are poorly connected. Effective paragraphing is key to establishing flow, with each paragraph containing one observation or idea and the paragraphs being connected so that the end of one paragraph leads to the next.

Compared with reports (see below), the structure of an essay is comparatively straightforward. An essay contains the following sections:

- Introduction, where the reader is told what the aim of the essay is and what will be covered in it
- Main body: where the argument is presented (supported by sources of information)
- Conclusion: where the points made earlier are summarised and a conclusion is described (even if there is no definitive conclusion, which is often the case)

Reports

Reports are different from essays in that they communicate the results of research and tend not to use an essay-style argumentative framework. The structure of reports is broadly similar (although, again, this may vary by discipline). Reports contain the following sections:

- Title (referring to all elements of the research)
- Abstract or summary
- Introduction and background literature review: this is where the rationale for the research is presented. This leads to the research aim or question
- Methods: this is where the student describes how they answered their research question
- Results: this is where findings are presented using words, tables, graphs and images
- Discussion: this summarises findings, discusses the limitations of the research and makes recommendations. A brief conclusion sometimes appears after the discussion

Sub-headings are used in reports, and the writing style is to-the-point. Appendices (supplementary text or figures not included in the main body of the report, often for reasons of space) can be useful to help you make sense of something in the report. For example, if you were writing a report about the effectiveness of different types of diabetes medication, you wouldn't necessarily have space in the report to describe technical aspects of the medication—such as the main chemical components—but these details could be included in an appendix).

Activity 2.2: Identify a report

Identify a health and social care report and look at its structure. Can you see how this is different from an essay? Does the report include appendices? What aspect of the report do these relate to?

Presentations

Presentations, whether done as a group or individually, often create anxiety for students, especially those who are nervous about public speaking. However, it's worth developing presentation skills because it's an important activity not only in education but also in the workplace. Presentations can help build confidence in even the shyest student and develop team-working skills, especially where a group of students are required to work together to give a presentation.

A presentation is, above all, an act of storytelling. In H&SC, the story will often be about a health condition, a form of treatment or an aspect of practice, and even if these topics appear to be rather unexciting topics to tell a story about, a well-developed and effectively delivered presentation can make even the most mundane issue engaging.

A mistake that many students often make when asked to give a presentation is that they go straight to Microsoft PowerPoint and start typing in text or copying and pasting images. A presentation will be far more effective if you develop a script first (although this does not need to written out in full). General tips and other 'top tips' for effective presentations are provided in Panel 2.3.

Panel 2.3: Top tips for effective presentations

1. Decide what kind of story you want to tell: Do this before you start structuring and designing the presentation
2. Know your audience: Make sure your presentation is appropriate for the audience
3. Structure the presentation with care: Presentations have a beginning, middle and end
4. Pay attention to design: If you are using PowerPoint or similar platforms, don't include too much text on the slides and be careful with strong or bold colours (such as red or black)
5. Practise, practise and practise some more: This will help you gain command of the presentation
6. Manage presentation nerves: Practise deep breathing and positive visualisation
7. Feel in control of the environment: Visit the room where you will present beforehand, ensure you know how to work the lighting, computer, etc. If you are delivering the presentation online, then be sure you are familiar with the technology and how to upload the slides
8. Interact with the audience: Make eye contact with the members of the audience (although don't hold their gaze for *too* long)
9. Be prepared for any questions: You don't have to know the answers to all questions asked; it's fine to tell a questioner you will get back to them
10. Reflect on what worked and what didn't work so well: This will help you develop your presentation skills. Don't be hard on yourself if the presentation didn't go as well as expected. This is a learning opportunity

---

Activity 2.3: Watch a TED talk

Watch a technology, entertainment and design (TED) talk. TED is a non-profit organisation that aims to spread ideas. It does this primarily through its TED talks; high-quality talks on a variety of topics (health, society, technology, personal growth, etc.). You can find a wide range of these on YouTube or at www.ted.com/. Choose one video and, after watching it, make a list of what makes it an interesting and engaging talk.

Case studies

A case study is an in-depth, anonymised examination of one person (or a group of people) or a company or organisation (such as a hospital). In H&SC, the case will usually be a patient (or possibly a group of patients) and will include discussion of all aspects of a case's social and medical history. Case studies are often used in reflective essays (so, students' accounts 'pivot' around their experience of interaction with one person). Case studies can be powerful: it's interesting to learn about one person and salient aspects of their life and to use this to illustrate a theory, idea or some aspect of learning, but special care should be taken when selecting a case. It's important to select the right case study for the assignment, one that is memorable or thought-provoking and can help illuminate your observations.

Case studies are widely used in research, although they are considered one of the less reliable research designs. Cottrell (2019) notes that one of the limitations of case studies is that they are based on one person or organisation, and the findings are not necessarily generalisable (so, they cannot be applied to a wider population). Similarly, she also advises that care must be taken when developing general rules from only one case study.

Examinations (including objective structured clinical examinations)

Most students are familiar with exams, as examinations are the main form of assessment at GCSE/'O' level and at 'A' level. These assignments are taken under exam conditions (meaning that they are timed, completed in silence and interaction with others is forbidden). Multiple choice questions are frequently used in examinations. This is where learners are given several possible choices to a question.

Objective structured clinical examinations (OSCEs) are a widely used form of practical examination in H&SC. They are used for clinical modules such as those focused on the management of medicines. Students undertaking OSCEs are presented with clinical scenarios at several different 'stations', and they must demonstrate competence in dealing with each scenario. Actors or models are often used in OSCEs, but training 'dolls' are also commonplace. You can see an image of an OSCE below.

Instructional or command verbs

Once you understand what kind of assignment you are being asked to write, you then need to examine the assignment task itself. This entails scrutinising the instructional or command verbs. The command words include 'describe', 'evaluate', 'summarise', 'compare' and 'critique', and these indicate what you should do.

Activity 2.4: Look at instructional verbs

Look at the list of instructional verbs developed by the University of Leeds (2022) at https://library.leeds.ac.uk/downloads/download/45/using_the_right_instructional_verbs. Can you see how these are all different (sometimes subtly so)?

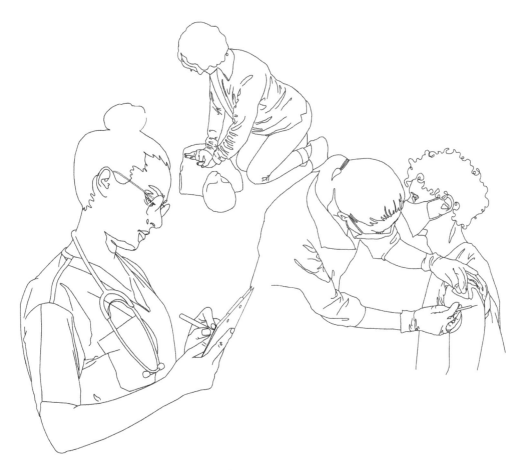

Figure 2.2 An objective structured clinical examination in process
Image credit: Tamsin Arai Drake

Pay special attention to the instructional verb. If you are asked to 'critique', for example, but you only 'describe', then your work is likely to be considered too descriptive and lacking depth. Similarly, if you are asked to 'illustrate' a concept (often done by reference to a practice experience in H&SC), but you only 'define', then the marker will likely comment on this, and it may affect your grade. See panel 2.4 for more information about instructional verbs.

Panel 2.4: Important note about instructional verbs

Some assignment tasks contain more than one instructional verb. See this essay task, for example: 'Describe the main steps in the founding of the NHS and examine the drivers for its creation'.

   Note that the student is first being asked to 'describe' and then to 'examine'. Description is relatively straightforward; the aim here is to be clear about what you are describing so that the reader will understand it. 'Examine' requires exploring something in greater depth, going beyond description. In this case, the student is being asked to examine the drivers (the forces) behind the creation of the NHS.

Instructional verbs can also be found in learning outcomes. What are these? These are the skills and knowledge a student should have to demonstrate once they have completed the module or programme.

Planning

As soon as you have read (and re-read) the assignment brief, you should start planning your assignment.

   Effective time management is key to meeting submission deadlines. Practitioner students are different from 'traditional' students in terms of the available time they have to complete assignments. H&SC students who are in the workplace for 4 days in a week and in the university for 1 day (as most apprentices are) do not have the luxury of procrastination; busy practitioners have no choice but to plan carefully if they are to submit their assignments on time. How this is done will be unique for each student. It may mean 'divvying' up tasks into manageable 'chunks' first, followed by identifying the information or other resources needed for each chunk of activity. Then each chunk could be allocated a rough estimate of time needed to complete it. Always keep the deadline in mind and avoid submitting work at the last minute. Don't forget that you need time to edit and proofread the edited work.

   Once you have an idea of what time you need, you can give some thought to the final submission and its structure. At this stage, though, you are still in the planning phase and still working out what needs to be done and by when.

Researching: finding and thinking

The second stage is about finding and assessing information, reading and making notes, thinking critically and formulating ideas. This is a creative stage where you draw on others' research, collate the findings from this research and 'synthesise' the ideas contained therein. What does 'synthesise' mean? It means combining information from different sources.

Identifying and evaluating academic resources

This is discussed in detail in chapter 3, so this topic will be only briefly covered here. In brief, it's imperative that you draw on reliable, academic resources for your assignment.

Avoid going straight to Google to identify resources. Instead, use academic resources such as the search engine Google Scholar and academic databases. The subject librarian at your institution is the authority on the academic databases the university has access to and will be able to guide you. The librarian also knows the best way to extract the information you need from these databases. (See chapter 3 for information on how to conduct a search strategy—this is where resources such as academic databases are searched to identify resources you need for your work).

Once you've identified resources for your assignment, you then need to consider carefully if the resource is reliable or not. A widely used test is the *CRAAP test*. This was developed by a librarian (Blakeslee 2004) to help students decide if a source of information is reliable or credible. See Figure 2.3 for more information about the *CRAAP test*.

Activity 2.5: Apply the CRAAP test

Apply the CRAAP test to an information source. This can be anything you like—a book, report or website. You can use the questions at https://libguides.cmich.edu/web_research/craap to help you with this task.

Websites are often less reliable than other sources of information. Look at the use of the CRAAP test in relation to two websites at https://libguides.cmich.edu/web_research/examples

---

Peer reviewed journal papers

In academia, the peer reviewed journal paper is one of the most important sources of information. Peer reviewed journal papers are articles that have been examined by experts in the field and subjected to scrutiny with regard to the methodology used, the presentation of findings as well as the contribution that the paper makes to the existing body of research. The kinds of questions peer reviewers might ask while reviewing the paper are as follows:

- Research design: does the study provide a strong rationale for the choice of research design? Is the design clearly described? Is the design appropriate for the research question?
- Data collection methods: are these methods described in sufficient detail? What data collection tools were used?
- Sampling: what is the sample size? How were research participants recruited?
- Data analysis: how robust is the data analysis? Are the steps in the analytic procedure described?
- Research ethics: does the study present ethical challenges? Was ethical approval secured?

Depending on the reviewers' assessment, journal papers may be accepted for publication, accepted with revisions or rejected outright.

CURRENCY
THE TIMELINESS
OF THE INFORMATION

- How recently was the information published?
- Has the information been revised or updated, and when was this?
- Is the information up-to-date or no longer relevant for your subject?
- Can all links still be accessed?

RELEVANCE
THE IMPORTANCE
OF THE INFORMATION
FOR YOUR NEEDS

- Does the information appropriately address your topic?
- What readership has been written for?
- Is the information written at an appropriate level?
- When selecting a source, how many other sources have been considered?

AUTHORITY
THE SOURCE OF
THE INFORMATION

- Do you know who the author, publisher or source is?
- Does the author have credentials or affiliations available, are they qualified to write on the subject?
- Is contact information given, such as an e-mail address or publisher?
- Does the author or source correspond with the URL?

ACCURACY
THE TRUTHFULNESS,
RELIABILITY AND
CORRECTNESS
OF THE CONTENT

- What is the source of the information? Has it been reviewed? Can it be verified by another source?
- Does evidence support the information?
- Can you detect bias or agenda?
- Is the language free from spelling, grammar or other typographical errors?

PURPOSE
THE REASON THAT
THE INFORMATION EXISTS

- Are the purpose and intentions of the authors clear?
- Is the information factual, or could it be an opinion or have an alternative agenda?
- Does it appear to be written from an unbiased and objective point of view?
- Can you detect the presence of bias? This could be personal, cultural, political, religious or institutional?

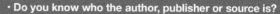

Figure 2.3 CRAAP test
Image credit: Tamsin Arai Drake, adapted from Blakeslee: (2004)

Peer review is not a perfect process; mistakes still happen. One of the most egregious examples of this is the Wakefield scandal. In 1998, Dr Andrew Wakefield's paper reporting a possible link between the measles, mumps and rubella (MMR) vaccine and autism in children was published in the highly prestigious medical journal *The Lancet*. However, his study was subsequently found to contain serious methodological and ethical flaws (including Dr Wakefield's failure to disclose conflicts of interest). The paper was eventually retracted, but Dr Wakefield's findings were reported in the popular press, which led to a reduction in the uptake of the MMR vaccine over several years. (See Deer (2020) for more information about the scandal.)

Notwithstanding the Wakefield affair, because journal papers are subject to quality appraisal by experts, this type of scholarly output is generally regarded as a reliable source of information, and you are advised to draw on journal papers for your assignments.

Reading and making notes

Many students struggle with reading. Either they lose interest quickly, can't retain information or become distracted while reading. It's also quite common for students to worry about their reading speed or to feel overwhelmed by the amount of reading they need to complete for their course.

There's no one way to read effectively; much depends on the learner, their skills, the text they are reading (for example, documents with documents containing statistical data or complex technical information usually need slow and careful reading) and the reason they are reading (is the learner engaging in background reading? Or is the text being read as a core reading and important for an assignment?)

Various tips and strategies have been proposed to help students to improve their reading skills. See Panel 2.5 for a brief overview of these tips and strategies.

Panel 2.5: Reading tips and strategies

- You don't have to read everything the same way—sometimes, it's appropriate to read a text briefly, whereas other texts may need a greater level of concentration and time
- If you are reading online, then use the full-screen mode or increase the zoom intensity on the page
- Whether reading online or a hard copy of a text, take regular breaks to prevent eye strain and tiredness
- Make time to read
- Three common techniques for reading are *scan-reading* (looking over a text quickly to identify the information needed), *skimming* (reading something quickly to get the 'gist' of it) and *deeper reading* (reading in detail and depth)

Take notes as you read (see below)—be careful to identify all information sources so that you don't lose track of where the information was found.

Activity 2.6: What helps when you are reading?

What is your experience of reading? Do you struggle to find the time and space to read? Do you read better in the morning or evening? Make a list of all the things that help you when you are reading.

Whatever strategy you use to help you with your reading, if you don't understand something you've just read, and you've re-read it several times, then it's a good idea to set the text to one side and do something else instead. Go for a walk, made a drink or move around. Cottrell (2019) writes that 'Just re-reading many times isn't usually helpful because …The brain is conditioned to 'zone out' when it encounters situations or material it recognises as familiar. It switches off to information it finds less stimulating or 'redundant'. Feed it a new angle' (p.244).

Note taking

You will be expected to take notes while you are studying, either in the classroom (whether online or real world) or during your reading. The Open University (2021) observes that taking notes can help you to '…improve your understanding by making you convert difficult ideas into your own words, prepare for writing fuller and better-connected arguments in your essays, be more focused and time-efficient during your exam revision period [and] assess your own progress as you study'. Note taking is also an important skill because, if done correctly, it helps you keep track of the information sources you cite in your work (and thus reduces the chances of unintentionally plagiarising; see below for more information about this concept).

As with reading, there's no one way to take notes and what works for one learner may not work for another. You should find a note-taking technique that works for you, and you may find that you use more than one, depending on the circumstances.

Activity 2.7: Read about note-taking techniques

Go to Open University (2021) resource on note taking at https://help.open.ac.uk/notetaking-techniques. Read the different techniques discussed. Which one do you prefer?

Critical thinking and formulating ideas

It was observed earlier that the 'researching' stage of the process of completing your work (and using a range of study skills while doing so) is a creative stage. Once you've identified the information you need for your work, assessed it to ensure it's appropriate for your assignment and made detailed notes, you then must arrange the information to make sense of it. This is where critical thinking skills really matter.

What do we mean by 'critical thinking'? Egan (2019) draws on Halpern (2003) definition of critical thinking as: '…the use of those cognitive skills or strategies that increase the probability of a desirable outcome. It is used to describe thinking that is purposeful, reasoned and goal directed' and observes that this definition: '… helps us to conceptualise critical thinking as being less about banging our fists on the table in an argument and more about *engaging in smart, thoughtful consideration*. It suggests an approach to thinking about different situations that is practical and outcome oriented' (p.26, emphasis added).

How can learners best engage in critical thinking? There are many resources aimed at students to help them develop this skill—too many to discuss here—and there are many scholarly theories about the nature of critical thinking and its development. Bloom's taxonomy (Bloom *et al.* 1956) is one of the most famous theories of learning. You can see the six categories of learning in Figure 2.4.

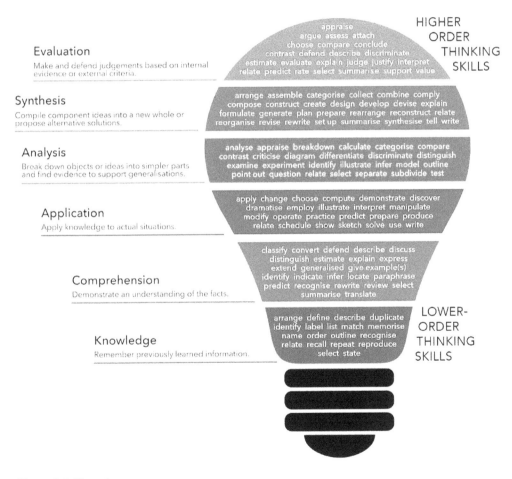

Figure 2.4 Bloom's taxonomy

Image credit: Tamsin Arai Drake, adapted from: Armstrong (2010)

All levels of this model are important—from simple recall of basic facts at the bottom to production of new work at the top. Learners (especially on foundation courses) often can't conceive of ever developing the upper-most skills, or even some of those skills below.

During an academic career, these skills will grow (especially as the student's submitted work become more proficient and higher grades are attained), but what is crucial to this development is the movement from description to analysis. It's quite common for academic staff to write expressions such as 'this is overly descriptive' or 'a deeper level of analysis is warranted' . These terms (and ones like them) are especially deployed in the marking of reflective essays (see Panel 2.2 on 'argumentative framework in essays' above), which usually require a description of the event or experience to be reflected on (most reflective frameworks include a specific description stage. See Gibbs (1988), for example). Importantly, for a 'deep' reflection to be demonstrated, the reflector must progress through stages such as 'analysis' and 'evaluation'. If there is too much description and not enough analysis, the reflection will likely not attract a high grade.

A good first step to developing critical thinking skills is to adopt a generally sceptical attitude to everything you read, hear and see. Question everything and be prepared to reject an argument if it seems flimsy or the evidence for it is not robust. (Of course, you must then create a cogent, evidence-based argument of your own).

Writing up: putting it all together

Academic writing

It's quite common for even the best prepared student to flounder when they write up their findings. This is understandable; it can be daunting to write in an academic style, especially if (as noted earlier) this is a new skill or a student has been out of education for a long time. Yet, learners who develop effective writing skills while at university are acquiring or honing a key transferable skill, one that will last a lifetime, so this skill should be encouraged and carefully nurtured at every opportunity. As McMillan and Weyers (2012) write:

> Writing is something that will not be confined to your university days... your ability to use the transferable skill of writing will mark you out as a competent communicator of facts and opinions. In your professional life, in all sorts of contexts and for all sorts of purposes, you will draw on the training you receive at university in presenting your ideas effectively on paper. Thus, writing well is an integral facet of the skills set that you take away with you from the university experience (p.3).

There are well established conventions governing academic writing and a great deal of help for learners in most colleges and universities. There are also many books and book chapters on this subject. One of the most accessible of these is Cottrell (2019). She refers to the 'Stylistic conventions for academic writing' as characterised by the use of

- Formal English: slang and colloquialisms (everyday expressions such as 'on the other hand' or 'at the end of the day') should be avoided. Abbreviations and contractions (for example, don't, 'shouldn't) should not be used

- Clear sentences: ensure that the text is understandable and avoid long, convoluted sentences. The language should be concise and to-the-point
- Specialist vocabulary: Cottrell (2019) advises noting how such terms are introduced in books and articles before using them in your work
- Impersonal and objective language: the first person ('I') should not be used. Instead, use terms such as 'the data show' or 'the evidence points to'. Subjective words such as 'disaster' or 'pleasant' should not be avoided
- Cautious tone: scholars need to be careful about 'backing themselves into a corner' with bold statements, so terms expressing a lack of certainty ('the data appear to', 'the findings may', 'it is apparently the case') are commonplace in academic literature
- Absence of advice for the reader: Cottrell (2019)l advises the avoidance of questions aimed at readers or telling readers what to think or do ('we need to reform community care')

Activity 2.8: Watch Queen's University Belfast academic writing style workshop

Queen's University Belfast has created an excellent 15-minute video on academic writing conventions. This can be accessed at www.youtube.com/watch?v=yi5tld98 ePE&t=181s
Watch and take notes.

Referencing and avoiding plagiarism

Most higher education institutions have an academic misconduct policy. This describes how academic misconduct is defined and what the penalties are for infringements of the policy. Academic misconduct is an umbrella term for several behaviours and activities, some relevant for research active staff and some for students. Among the latter, academic misconduct is associated primarily with plagiarism, which involves using someone else's work or ideas in an assignment without full acknowledgement by the writer. This is often unwitting—a consequence of failure to cite sources appropriately and general poor academic practice (not keeping a list of sources cited).

The key message here is: keep a note of all sources used in your assignment, and be sure to cite accordingly. It is better to over-cite than to under-cite (and risk being accused of plagiarism). Be sure to follow your university or college's referencing style (these vary enormously).

Occasionally, plagiarism occurs because of poor paraphrasing. What is paraphrasing? This is where someone else's ideas are expressed in your own words. Paraphrasing is not as easy as it seems. Many students paraphrase by simply moving the order of words around or by using synonyms (the so-called 'linguistic approach'). This is often a mistake. The use of synonyms, in particular, can render a text gobbledygook. Learners who speak English as a second or additional language should be advised to avoid the use of synonyms. It's not always possible to replace one word with another in the English language because words can have many meanings. For example, this sentence: 'There is an escalating quantity of people who have asthma in south London' is likely to sound 'not quite right' to a native English speaker (although the overall sense of the sentence can be understood). In this sentence, the original term for 'escalating quantity' was almost certainly 'an increase in numbers or rates' or similar, but 'escalating quantity' does not have the same 'ring' and sounds clumsy.

A far better approach to paraphrasing is to read a text, make your own notes and then attempt to write in your own words what you have read (it's a good idea to step aside from the text after making notes—go for a walk, make a cup of tea—and then return to writing in your own words). See Panel 2.6 below.

Panel 2.6: Steps in a notes and memory-based approach to paraphrasing

- Read the text
- Make notes
- Close the text (and, preferably, do something else)
- Return to the text (after a break)
- Rewrite—in your own words and based on memory and notes—a summary of the original text.

Activity 2.9: Read your institution's academic misconduct policy

Read your institution's academic misconduct policy. Make a note of how plagiarism is defined and what the penalties are for it.

Proofreading

The final activity we will examine here is proofreading. What is proofreading? It's where the document you are working on (essay, report, etc.) is checked for errors and whether it's referenced appropriately. It's common for students to forget this stage (or, more usually, fail to allocate enough time to complete this task thoroughly). It's a good idea to proofread the document more than once and, also, to ask a fellow student to check for any unnoticed mistakes.

Once the document has been proofread, a useful activity involves checking the final submission against the learning outcomes specified for the module and assignment. Remember, these are the skills, knowledge and competencies that a student should be able to demonstrate after completion of the module. Most assignment briefs contain learning outcomes. You can see an example of typical learning outcomes for a level 5 service improvement project module in Panel 2.7. Pay especial attention to the verbs (identify, collect, analyse, etc.)

Panel 2.7: Typical learning outcomes—example of a level 5 service improvement project module

- Identify a salient, small-scale and low-cost service improvement idea and present a cogent rationale for the selection of this idea
- Collect and analyse audit data in the workplace
- Explain project planning processes
- Implement a service improvement project
- Demonstrate critical awareness of ethical, logistical and other factors affecting project implementation
- Communicate effectively through a poster presentation and a verbal defence.

Dealing with feedback

Summative and formative feedback

Students often confuse these two forms of feedback. While both are important, they are fundamentally different in terms of the nature of the feedback given: formative work is assessed informally (that is, a grade is not awarded), while summative work is allocated a grade. Formative feedback may be given verbally or in written form, whereas summative feedback is nearly always written (it can also be verbal).

It's quite common for learners not to complete formative assignments or not to take the feedback from them seriously because no formal grade is awarded. This is a mistake; completing formative assignments and getting feedback is an excellent way to improve your summative assignment.

Using feedback effectively

Activity 2.10: How do you deal with feedback?

Think about how you deal with summative feedback. If the grade you've been awarded for a piece of summative work is not as high as you expected, how does this make you feel? Do you feel 'spurred on' to do better next time? Or does it make you feel dejected?

As discussed earlier, many H&SC students are mature learners and have been out of the education system for many years and may therefore lack confidence. They often struggle with some academic skills (writing, critiquing, referencing, etc.) and can feel despondent if the grade for their work is not as high as expected (or if their work doesn't attain a pass grade).

A great deal has been written about how academic staff can provide meaningful feedback. Arguably, less attention has been given to the impact of feedback on students' emotions and motivation. Hill *et al.* (2021), however, point to a growing interest in this topic and, in their analysis of student response to summative feedback (defined as: '...as high-stakes, stressful episodes by students, which directly expose their capabilities as learner...' (p.295)), maintain that students' emotional response to summative feedback plays a significant role in determining how they receive and act on feedback.

Their findings demonstrate that feedback comments perceived as negative were difficult to receive by students and '...drew out particularly powerful emotions...' (p.310). The words and phrases that participants reported in this study–'it's kind of like a punch to yourself–it stings', I just keep beating myself up about it' 'It's completely crushing'–illustrate this very well.

If you don't get the grade you'd hoped, or tutor feedback is not wholly positive, then learn from the experience. It's not a reflection on you or your personal qualities; you simply didn't meet the threshold for passing that assignment, or you didn't attain as high a grade as hoped.

Summary

In this chapter, we explored selected key study skills. The essential study skills fall (broadly speaking) in three areas. 'Preparing' is about understanding the task you are being asked to undertake, especially in terms of the assignment type. It's also about planning the assignment. 'Researching' is the creative and intellectual phase when you identify and evaluate information for your assignment, make notes and formulate ideas. The final phase, 'Writing up', focuses on the actual writing up of your findings, editing and proofreading. Developing the skills discussed in this chapter will help you to become an autonomous learner: someone who is self-motivated and able to direct themselves.

Box 2.4: Key learning points

- The essential study skills fall into three areas: 'Preparing', focused on understanding the task you are being asked to undertake and planning the assignment; 'Researching', the creative phase involving formulating ideas and 'Writing up'
- To attain deep learning, students should engage with, and complete, all three stages
- It's important to understand the distinction between essays, report and other types of assignments
- Peer reviewed journal papers are the most important scholarly output
- As you progress through higher education, you will develop your critical thinking skills. This involves going beyond description in your assignments
- Academic writing is characterised by the use of language that is formal, scholarly and free of colloquial expressions.

References

ARMSTRONG, P., 2010. *Bloom's Taxonomy*. Vanderbilt University Center for Teaching [viewed 17 August 2022]. Available from: https://cft.vanderbilt.edu/guides-sub-pages/blooms-taxonomy/

BLAKESLEE, S., 2004. The CRAAP Test. *LOEX quarterly*, 31(3), 4 [viewed 17 August 2022]. Available from: https://commons.emich.edu/loexquarterly/vol31/iss3/4.

BLOOM, B. S. *et al.*, 1956. *Taxonomy of educational objectives: The classification of educational goals. Vol. Handbook I: Cognitive domain.* New York: David McKay Company.

COTTRELL, S., 2019. *The study skills handbook.* 5th ed. London: Macmillan International Higher Education: Red Globe Press.

COWEN, M., P. MAIER and G. PRICE, 2013. *Study skills for nursing and healthcare students.* Electronic ed. London: Pearson Education Limited.

DEER, B., 2020. *The doctor who fooled the world: Science, deception, and the war on vaccines.* London: Scribe UK.

EGAN, A., 2019. *Confidence in critical thinking: Developing learners in higher education.* Abingdon, Oxon: Routledge.

GIBBS, G., 1988. *Learning by doing: A guide to teaching and learning methods.* Further Education Unit. Oxford Polytechnic: Oxford.

HALPERN, D. F., 2003. *Thought and knowledge: An introduction to critical thinking* 4th ed. Mahwah, NJ: Lawrence Erlbaum.

HILL, J. *et al.*, 2021. Exploring the emotional responses of undergraduate students to assessment feedback: Implications for instructors. *Teaching and learning inquiry*, 9(1), 294-318. https://doi.org/10.20343/teachlearninqu.9.1.20

McMILLAN, K. and J. WEYERS, 2012. *The study skills book.* 3rd ed. Harlow, Essex: Pearson Education Limited.

NURSING AND MIDWIFERY COUNCIL, 2018. *Nursing and midwifery standards of proficiency for nursing associates* [viewed 7 January 2023]. Available from: www.nmc.org.uk/globalassets/sitedocuments/standards-of-proficiency/nursing-associates/nursing-associates-proficiency-standards.pdf

OPEN POLYTECHNIC, 2022. *Step-by-step guide to tackling assignments* [viewed 15 August 2022]. Available from: www.openpolytechnic.ac.nz/current-students/study-tips-and-techniques/assignments/step-by-step-guide-to-tackling-assignments/

OPEN UNIVERSITY, 2021. *Note-taking techniques* [viewed 7 January 2023]. Available from: https://help.open.ac.uk/notetaking-techniques

UNIVERSITY OF LEEDS, 2022. *Using the right instructional verbs* [viewed 17 August 2022]. Available from: https://library.leeds.ac.uk/downloads/download/45/using_the_right_instructional_verbs

3 Research, the research 'basics' and evidence-based practice

Lisa Arai

Box 3.1: Contents

- Introduction
- What is research and research evidence?
- Research in health and social care
- Research methodology: A brief overview
- Designing a small-scale research project
- Evidence-based practice: What is it and how is it done?
- Research literacy and using research evidence in your assignments

---

Box 3.2: Learning outcomes

By the end of this chapter, you should be able to

- Define research and research evidence
- Identify examples of health and social care research
- Demonstrate basic knowledge of research methodology
- Engage with evidence-based practice
- Describe the stages of a research project
- Demonstrate knowledge of how to use research in your assignments.

Box 3.3: Keywords

- Research evidence
- Research methodology
- Quantitative research
- Qualitative research
- Primary research
- Secondary research
- Critical appraisal

DOI: 10.4324/9781003198338-4

Introduction

Students don't usually engage in research 'proper' until level 6, when they complete a dissertation of five to 10,000 words. However, foundation degree students are required to draw on research evidence to support their assignments and to critique and synthesise research findings. Practitioner students are also required to be 'evidence-based' in their practice. This central concept in health and social care (H&SC) practice will be considered here.

To perform well, foundation degree students need a basic understanding of research and research evidence, knowledge of how to locate and identify research evidence and understanding of how to use research evidence in assignments and in practice. These activities are discussed in this chapter. We also examine what the terms 'research' and 'research evidence' mean, consider how research evidence can be used to inform H&SC practice, discuss how to design a small-scale research project, consider the application of research evidence to practice and briefly explore the use of research in your assignments.

What is research and research evidence?

Activity 3.1: What does 'research' mean?

Before we explore what research means, can you define 'research' in one or two sentences?

According to the Oxford Dictionary, 'research' is defined as: 'The systematic investigation into, and study of, materials and sources in order to establish facts and reach new conclusions'. Note the elements of this definition—'systematic', 'study of materials and sources', 'facts' and 'conclusions'—all of which define the main features of research.

The National Health Service (NHS) Research Authority's definition of research is that it is: '... the attempt to derive generalisable or transferable ... new... knowledge to answer or refine relevant questions with scientifically sound methods (NHS Research Authority 2021). The reference to 'generalisable' and 'transferable' is about the applicability of research more broadly; can research findings be generalised to a wider population? This important concept is explored in Panel 3.1.

Panel 3.1: Generalisability

Generalisability refers to the extent to which research findings can be generalised from the sample to a larger population. Where sample sizes are small (as is often the case with qualitative research—see below), generalisability may be limited. In the 'limitations' section of a journal paper or report, researchers usually discuss the extent to which their findings are generalisable. For example, in Ni *et al.*'s study of barriers and levers to data quality of electronic clinical research health records in

China, 19 research participants in four hospitals in Beijing were interviewed. The authors note that: 'The limitations of this study include that the participants were recruited from four hospitals in Beijing and that the generalisability of the findings may be limited because of the small sample size' (Ni *et al.* 2019, p.6).

Once research has been conducted and published, it becomes 'research evidence'. Another term you might hear is 'research literature'. These terms refer to outputs written by academics and others (such as policymakers). One of the most important sources of research evidence are papers published in academic journals (although research evidence is also published in books, reports and oral presentations). Academic journals are significant sources because they publish research in their respective field and most journal papers are peer-reviewed. See Panel 3.2.

Panel 3.2: The peer review process

When an author submits his or her paper to an academic journal, it is then disseminated to external experts who are asked to give their opinion as to the paper's overall quality, the reliability of the methods used and its suitability to the journal. Peer reviewers are usually provided with a list of questions to consider when appraising the submission by the journal's editorial team (see chapter 2 for more information). Reviewers then recommend that the paper is either accepted (with or without amendments) or rejected.

Research in health and social care

Like other academic disciplines, H&SC has its own academic journals where research is reported. There are many journals in this field and related fields (such as public health).

Activity 3.2: Identify a health and social care journal

Identify a health and social care journal by typing the words 'health and social care' and 'journal' in a search engine (such as Google). What journals did you identify?

In H&SC, high-quality and reliable research is of paramount importance. Research underpins all aspects of care provided to patients, clients and service users. Comprehensive research, for example, about the size and characteristics of a population, is necessary for H&SC services to meet local health needs. H&SC research often focuses on people's experiences of living with a condition (diabetes, asthma or human immunodeficiency virus) so that practitioners can best meet the needs of patients. There is a large body of research on the most effective way to provide specialised treatment and interventions to individuals living with, or at risk of, conditions such as cardiovascular disease. To treat these patients, there is an ongoing need for high-quality research.

H&SC academic journals report different types of research findings and can include papers not reporting research findings, such as commentaries or editorials. It can be bewildering when you first start reading academic journals. You may struggle to understand the aim of the paper, the methods used and what the results mean. This is understandable; this is a complex area and, to understand academic papers, some knowledge of research methodology is necessary. This is what we will explore in the sections below.

Research methodology: a brief overview

Foundation degree students don't usually need to understand *everything* about research methodology because (as noted above) they don't undertake a research project as part of their degree. However, for the reasons described earlier, and especially if you decide to study beyond foundation level or become involved with a research project at work (such as a drugs trial or service improvement project), it would be useful to know the research 'basics'. What are these?

Primary and secondary research

The types of research papers you read in journals fall (largely) into two categories: papers reporting findings from primary research and papers reporting findings from secondary research.

Primary research refers to research wherein original or new data have been collected (where, for example, there is little research on a specific topic). Secondary research refers to research wherein no original data are collected, but the research uses existing sources of data (the data created by primary researchers).

Many students at levels 4 and 5 (and even at level 6) do not engage in primary research because it presents significant ethical, practical and logistical challenges (the latter are briefly discussed below; see chapter 11 for a description of ethics).

Activity 3.3: Identify two papers

Using a search engine such as Google Scholar, identify a paper reporting primary findings and one reporting secondary findings.

Quantitative and qualitative data

In H&SC research, two main types of data are collected and analysed: quantitative and qualitative. Quantitative data are statistical and are collected when measuring or counting phenomena. Qualitative data are words (they can also be images and audio—any data that are not easily counted) and are more exploratory and collected to understand people's motivations and experiences. Qualitative data can be especially useful where quantitative research has demonstrated the existence of a problem and there is a need for a 'deep dive'.

Researchers collecting quantitative data aim to secure as large a sample size as possible and will often formulate a hypothesis (a prediction) to test their ideas. Sample size is less important for qualitative researchers because qualitative researchers do not necessarily seek to generalise their findings (see Panel 3.1 above).

Whether research is primary or secondary, quantitative or qualitative in nature (or both—mixed methods approaches are common) , these decisions are made at the research design stage. Once the (overall) design is finalised, the researcher must then decide how data will be collected and analysed.

Collection and analysis of data

In a primary research project, data are collected face-to-face (in the real world, online or by 'phone) in one-to-one interviews or focus groups. Data can also be collected using questionnaires or through observation. In a secondary project, other researchers' data and information are used.

A common type of research study is a systematic review. This is explored below but, briefly here, this is an authoritative, high-quality summary of the research evidence on a specific topic. Systematic reviews are useful for H&SC practitioners because all available research evidence on a specific issue is 'pooled' and summarised for use in practice.

Activity 3.4: Identify a systematic review

Using a search engine such as Google Scholar, identify a systematic review. Don't worry if you don't understand everything in the review; just make a note of the focus of the review, the methods used and the main findings.

Another type of secondary research is where existing data are re-analysed. This is called 'secondary analysis', and it can be done with either quantitative or qualitative data.

Once data are collected, they must then be analysed. Primary qualitative researchers often use thematic analysis. This widely used method of analysis is one of the most accessible analytic approaches and involves identifying codes (ideas or concepts) in raw qualitative data. Braun and Clarke's (2006) six steps in a thematic analysis approach is widely used. See Panel 3.3 below for a description of these steps.

Panel 3.3: Steps in a thematic analysis

- Familiarise yourself with the data
- Generate initial codes
- Search for themes
- Review themes
- Define and name themes
- Write up findings

Adapted from: Braun and Clarke (2006).

Quantitative data are analysed differently from qualitative data. The data are usually subjected to what's called a 'descriptive analysis', wherein summary statistics (mean, median, mode, range, etc.) are calculated. Statistical data can then be analysed further to explore relationships between variables (things that vary, such as gender, age, health status). The results of analysis of quantitative data are presented in tables, images and graphs.

These are the 'basics' of research design. Knowing this, how do you design a research project?

Designing a small-scale research project

The research cycle

Figure 3.1 shows the research cycle. These are the stages researchers necessarily pass through when conducting research.

Although this is a cycle, real-world research can often be a case of 'two steps forward, three steps back' as earlier steps are revisited, reviewed and possibly amended. Maybe the researcher realises that the original aim is not feasible or maybe data collection 'goes off' on an interesting tangent, taking him or her somewhere that hadn't been anticipated. Sometimes, a research project has to be revised because it wasn't very well designed in the first place. It is important to pay attention at the design stage and to consider all stages in the process carefully. We will now look at each of these steps.

Research question (what am I doing?)

At this stage, the researcher formulates a relevant and feasible research question. Most students start this process with a broad idea of what they are interested in and then they narrow down towards a focused question.

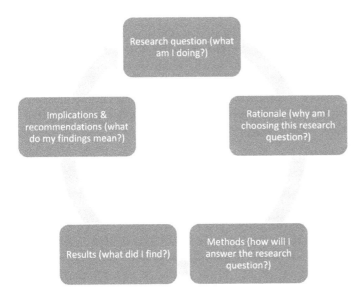

Figure 3.1 The research cycle
Created by: Lisa Arai

For example, a student with a general interest in metabolic disorders might decide to focus on type 2 diabetes (T2DM). However, this is still a big topic, one on which there is a large body of research, so the student then opts to focus on one group affected by T2DM—black and minority ethnic (BME) groups, for example, or one aspect of T2DM (diagnosis). The student's research question then becomes: 'What are the experiences of being diagnosed with T2DM among BME groups?' The student could even restrict their research to BME groups with T2DM in a specific place (the United Kingdom, London).

The aim and objectives derive from the research question. Students sometimes confuse these; aim relates to what you want to *do* or *achieve* in research and is the same as the research question but written as an aim, whereas objectives are focused on *how* you will achieve the project (Bowling 2014).

Rationale (why am I choosing this research question?)

The rationale is simply the reason why you are doing the research. In H&SC, it's relatively easy to create a rationale because of the focus on the prevention, or management of, chronic and other health conditions, and a case can usually be made for a condition or an issue being a problem or needing attention. Childhood obesity rates are increasing, for example, and, if not treated, childhood obesity can extend to obesity in adulthood. Asthma is a common chronic condition and, if not well managed, can lead to exacerbations and even death.

The strongest rationales are those that include consideration of the prevalence (frequency) of a condition or issue, discuss the impacts of the condition or issue (by referring to the harm to patient well-being, distress to families and loved ones, increased workload for H&SC staff and costs to healthcare systems) and describe policy initiatives to address the issue. It's important when developing the rationale to draw on the most recent data to support all statements.

Methods (how will I answer the research question?)

This is the stage of the research cycle where you describe how you will answer the research question. Research methodology was briefly considered earlier, so this topic will not be revisited here. However, it's important to note that this stage can be challenging for even the most experienced researchers. The researcher must choose one or more approaches and methods from a vast and complex array of methodological choices. The researcher is also limited by the more practical considerations of time, accessibility, costs and expertise.

A common problem for student researchers is ensuring that their projects can be completed in the time available. Primary research can be time-consuming and expensive. During the process of collecting data for the project, costs related to travel and accommodation may be incurred by the primary researcher. Qualitative researchers interviewing research participants typically record the interviews. These recorded interviews then need to be transcribed (where the spoken words are transformed into written ones). If a professional transcriber is employed, then this is an additional cost. A significant barrier to primary research is the willingness (or lack of) of would-be research participants to engage with the project. Some populations are considered 'hard to reach', like commercial sex workers or socially disadvantaged groups (Bonevski *et al.* 2014).

A student may want to interview healthcare workers as part of their research project, but it's not always easy to collect data from busy NHS employees (and ethical approval to do so can be onerous; see chapter 11). Somebody who doesn't like numbers would be ill advised to initiate research on establishing the prevalence of a condition because this kind of project would necessarily involve collection and analysis of statistical data (see chapter 12). Researchers engaged in secondary research can be constrained by the availability of secondary information on a topic.

The researcher is advised to identify the methodological approach and methods most appropriate for their project but needs to bear these practical considerations in mind.

Results (what did I find?)

This section is where the findings from the research endeavour are presented and usually involves the use of text, tables, images, graphs and figures. Exactly what type of analysis is presented depends on the nature of the research project—quantitative projects present findings in tables and graphs, and qualitative projects often report the analysis of research participants' views and opinions (in the form of 'themes'; see the section on thematic analysis).

Implications and recommendations (what do my findings mean?)

The final stage of the research cycle is where the researcher attempts to make sense of their findings and to think about what they mean for policy, practice and further research. All H&SC research projects make recommendations. In this field, we are interested in the application of our work more widely. Can the findings be utilised in the treatment of patients, for example? Do the findings have implications for policy? Importantly, would we recommend a change in practice as a result of our research endeavours? This is what we will look at in the sections below.

Evidence-based practice: what is it and how is it done?

Once research has been published in academic journals or elsewhere, it can then be used by H&SC practitioners who are required to adopt what's called an 'evidence-based' approach to the care of others. For example, the Nursing and Midwifery Council, the body that regulates nursing and midwifery in the United Kingdom, stipulates in its code of professional standards and behaviour that nurses, nursing associates and midwives must: '... make sure that any information or advice given is evidence based, including information relating to using any healthcare products or services' (Nursing and Midwifery Council 2018, p.7).

What is evidence-based practice (EBP)? Many definitions have been offered by commentators, but the one provided by Sackett *et al.* is widely accepted as the most significant one. For Sackett *et al.* (1996), evidence-based medicine is:

The conscientious, explicit and judicious use of current best practice in making decisions about the care of individual patients. The practice of evidence based medicine means integrating individual clinical expertise with the best available external clinical evidence from systematic research (p.71).

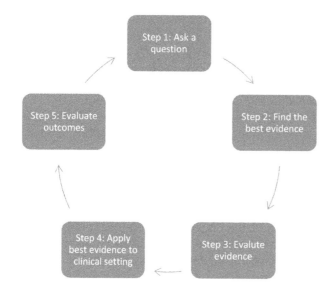

Figure 3.2 Five steps in evidence-based practice
Adapted from: Johnson (2008)

This definition specifically refers to the field of medicine, but this definition now has wider application and is used in areas beyond medicine, such as social policy and education.

Sackett *et al.* wrote that 'best practice' is about utilising the expertise of practitioners as well as drawing on 'evidence from systematic research.' Research evidence is, therefore, an essential component of EBP. Sackett *et al.* (1996, p.71) also pointed to the importance of patient values and preferences ('… thoughtful identification and compassionate use of individual patients' predicaments, rights and preferences in making clinical decisions about their care').

EBP has benefits for patients and service users as their care is informed by the latest research developments. EBP is also good for professionals; it can help in the development of professional knowledge and is an essential element in practitioners' career advancement strategies.

How can you 'do' EBP as a H&SC practitioner? This is what we will examine now.

Steps in the evidence-based practice process

There is a large body of work on EBP and many models and frameworks. One of the most widely used framework has five steps (Figure 3.2).

These steps are sometimes called the 'five As' (Hoffmann, Bennett and Del Mar 2017) and can be rewritten as:

- Ask the answerable question
- Acquire the best evidence to answer the question
- Appraise the evidence
- Apply the evidence
- Assess the outcome

We will look at each of these in detail.

Ask the answerable question

To identify relevant academic literature, the practitioner needs to develop a focused and refined research question, a point made earlier in this chapter.

The practitioner also needs to decide what kind of question he or she is asking. If the aim is to ascertain whether a particular clinical treatment works, for example, then this is an effectiveness-type question. The clinician might also be interested in peoples' experiences of receiving the treatment, as this is likely to significantly impact patient adherence. This kind of question is more likely to be answered with qualitative data.

There are several models and tools to aid researchers in the development of different types of question. See Panel 3.4 for an overview of two of these models.

Panel 3.4: Developing research questions using PICO and PIO

When developing effectiveness-type questions, a 'PICO' model can be used. PICO stands for:

- P = Population (patient, problem)
- I = Intervention (treatment)
- C = Comparison (control, comparator)
- O = Outcome

In the case of a question about the effectiveness of a new pharmacological treatment for the management of paediatric asthma exacerbation compared with an existing one, for example, the PICO might be expanded as:

- P = Paediatric asthma exacerbation/children with asthma who experience exacerbation
- I = New drug for the management of paediatric asthma exacerbation
- C = Existing drug for the management of paediatric asthma exacerbation
- O = More effective management of paediatric asthma exacerbation

The outcome in this example can be refined further by specifying what kind of outcome the researcher is interested in (reduction in hospital emergency admissions?)

The same question can be asked using a 'PIO' model. In this case, there is no comparator (so, the effectiveness of the new drug is not measured against any other treatment).

PIO can also be used with questions that are about people's experiences or views. In this case, PIO is:

- P = Population (patient, problem)
- I = Issue
- O = Outcome

These kinds of questions are often answered by speaking to people directly and collecting qualitative data. If a researcher is interested in children's experiences of being diagnosed with asthma, for example, PIO might be formulated as:

- P = Children with asthma
- I = Diagnosis of asthma
- O = Experiences

Acquire the best evidence

This step involves searching academic sources for information, especially electronic databases, to identify resources to draw on when answering the research question.

Before you search academic literature, you should identify any systematic reviews (or any other kind of review) on your topic. As noted above, these are reviews focused on a narrowly defined question and completed by strictly adhering to published guidelines. Systemic reviews are useful because they 'pool' all available research findings and summarise it. One place to search for systematic reviews is the Cochrane Database of Systematic Reviews (www.cochranelibrary.com/cdsr/about-cdsr).

Search strategies

The search strategy relates to the tools and techniques used to identify relevant research. Search strategies have at least three elements: what, where and how.

The 'what' aspect deals with the types of academic items (papers, books, reports, etc.) and inclusion criteria (the elements of an article or report that should be present in order for it to be used to answer the research question. A research question about older people's dementia care, for example, can only be answered by utilising information from papers or reports that report data on that issue).

The 'where' aspect refers to the resources used to identify academic items meeting the inclusion criteria. Contemporary search strategies use electronic databases identify items. There are other publicly available databases that can be used, including Google Scholar (https://scholar.google.co.uk/).

The 'how' aspect refers to techniques that can be used to search effectively and the speciality of librarians who are skilled in effective searching of databases. Most student researchers do need to have advanced search skills but would need to know the basics.

In most electronic databases, the search bar allows you to enter search terms ('children', 'older people', 'dementia' and 'obesity'). These are also known as 'keywords' and can be used with synonyms to widen the search, other limits (language, year of publication, etc.) and the use of Boolean operators such as 'AND', 'OR' or 'NOT'– 'AND' between search terms returns only records that contain all search terms. 'OR' between search terms returns all records that contain any of the search terms and 'NOT' between search terms returns only records that contain the first term and not the second.

Activity 3.5: Develop and execute a search strategy

You would almost certainly have engaged with electronic databases and other resources as part of your educational programme so the skills you need for this activity are not likely to be new to you. This activity will help you develop more structured and methodical ways to search for, and engage with, the research literature.

- First, think of a (broad) clinical problem or health topic you are interested in (childhood obesity, human immunodeficiency virus/acquired immunodeficiency syndrome, encouraging exercise in older people, etc.)
- Then create a research question using PICO or PIO
- Develop a search strategy. This means deciding: what you are searching for, where you are searching and how you are searching. You should decide what your inclusion criteria are (that is, what kind of evidence you will include). You should use two or more electronic databases and as many additional resources as you want. You should make a list of search terms you plan to use and consider using Boolean operators
- Run your search. This means entering the various search terms, limiting by year (if you want to) and recording your results.

Appraise the evidence

The third step of the EBP process where the evidence identified is evaluated. This process is also called 'critical appraisal' and is about assessing how methodologically robust research is. How can researchers critically appraise? There is extensive guidance on critical appraisal, and many tools have been developed to aid researchers. These are in the form of checklists. The Critical Appraisal Skills Programme (https://casp-uk.net/) checklists are among the most widely used.

Activity 3.6: Look at the Critical Appraisal Skills Programme checklists

Look at the Critical Appraisal Skills Programme checklists at https://casp-uk.net/ casp-tools-checklists/. Can you see that checklists have been developed for different types of studies (cohort studies, randomised controlled trials, etc.). What kinds of questions are asked in these checklists?

Apply the evidence

By this stage of the EBP process, the practitioner has identified a sample of research papers or other items meeting inclusion criteria from a literature search, has critically appraised those meeting inclusion criteria and he or she now has to apply the evidence. This involves consideration of how research findings can be utilised in real-world clinical settings, and it especially means thinking about the experiences of patients or service users who might be asked to engage with new forms of treatment or new approaches to their care. At this stage, we see the three elements of EBP working equally together. Johnson (2008) writes this step that it should: '... combine the new information [identi-fied from the literature search] with one's clinical experience *while paying attention to the patient's values*' (p.170, italicisation added).

Assess the outcome

The fifth and final step in the EBP process is about reviewing the effect of any changes in practice as a result of step 4. Further changes may be needed if the change in practice is not working as effectively as it could.

Research literacy and using research evidence in your assignments

Thus far, we have examined research and research design, considered how to develop a research project and explored the use of research as one element of EBP.

At foundation-level study, you are likely to need to demonstrate knowledge and understanding of these activities and, to some extent, be able to use them in your studies (this is especially true of skills including searching the literature). Whatever the demands of your programme, you must be research literate if you are to succeed on your course. What does this term mean?

There is no one definition of 'research literacy' and no one list of skills that demon-strate possession of it. At a minimum, it includes the following:

- Knowing what research is and how it's different from other information-seeking activities (for example, checking a bus timetable or engaging with consumer product reviews before a purchase)
- Understanding the 'basics' of research methodology and methods
- Possession of the necessary technical skills to complete a search of the research litera-ture using electronic databases and other resources
- Being able to navigate different types of scholarly outputs (journal papers, and aca-demic reports) and understanding the differences between them
- Developing critical appraisal skills so that the less methodologically reliable research can be separated from the more reliable one
- Being able to make sense of, and synthesise, often complex (and sometimes contra-dictory) research findings when constructing arguments
- Knowing when and where to seek help (from a librarian, for example)

In respect of the use of research evidence in your assignments, remember that citation of relevant research is paramount but it's also important to go beyond simple description when discussing findings.

Your tutor will notice when you discuss key methodological aspects of the research you are citing, especially in terms of its strengths and limitations (these are often related to sample size, problems with participant recruitment and inability to generalise findings). Your tutor will also notice when you make links across studies: how is this study different from the preceding one? In what way are the methods the same or different? What new conclusions have the authors drawn? How, as a collective body of research, do these contribute to my understanding of this topic? These kinds of skills demonstrate higher-level learning and will help you if you progress to study at level 6 or higher.

Summary

In this chapter, we defined research, examined its contribution to H&SC knowledge and practice and explored the research methodology 'basics'—the foundational ideas and theories underpinning research project design. All research projects progress through the research cycle, the stages of which include formulating a research question, describing the methods that will be used to answer the research question and presenting the findings. Research is utilised in the EBP process, but clinical judgement and patient values are equally important to this. All students need an elementary knowledge of research, research design and how to locate and make sense of research, as research evidence is drawn on in classroom and summative work. Developing these skills at levels 4 and 5 will help students equip for further learning at level 6 and above.

Box 3.4: Key learning points

- Research is a systematic investigation to establish facts and draw new conclusions
- Research in health and social care is necessary if the care needs of patients and service users are to be met
- There are a diverse range of research methodologies and methods. Research can be primary or secondary and qualitative or quantitative. It can also be mixed
- During the research endeavour, the researcher progresses through the stages of the research cycle, beginning from formulating a relevant and focused question to making recommendations
- High-quality research evidence is one element of evidence-based practice. Health and social care professionals are required to integrate the evidence with their own clinical judgement and patient values as part of this process
- Research literacy is essential for students to attain success on their educational programmes.

References

BONEVSKI, B. *et al.*, 2014. Reaching the hard-to-reach: A systematic review of strategies for improving health and medical research with socially disadvantaged groups. *BMC medical research methodology* , 14, 42. https://doi.org/10.1186/1471-2288-14-42

BOWLING, A., 2014. *Research methods in health: Investigating health and health services.* 4th ed. Maidenhead: Open University Press.

BRAUN, V. and V. CLARKE, 2006. Using thematic analysis in psychology. *Qualitative research in psychology*, 3(2), 77-101. https://doi.org/10.1191/1478088706qp063oa

HOFFMANN, T., S. BENNETT and C. DEL MAR, 2017. *Evidence-based practice across the health professions.* 3rd ed. Chatswood, NSW: Elsevier.

JOHNSON, C., 2008. Evidence-based practice in five simple steps. *Journal of manipulative and physiological therapeutics*, 31(3), 169-254. https://doi.org/10.1016/j.jmpt.2008.03.013

NHS RESEARCH AUTHORITY, 2021. *UK policy framework for health and social care research* [viewed 25 September 2022]. Available from: www.hra.nhs.uk/planning-and-improving-resea rch/policies-standards-legislation/uk-policy-framework-health-social-care-research/uk-policy-framework-health-and-social-care-research/

NI, K. *et al.*, 2019. Barriers and facilitators to data quality of electronic health records used for clinical research in China: A qualitative study. *BMJ open*, 9(7), e029314. https://doi.org/10.1136/bmjopen-2019-029314

NURSING AND MIDWIFERY COUNCIL, 2018. *Nursing and midwifery standards of proficiency for nursing associates* [viewed 17 August 2022]. London: NMC. Available from: www.nmc.org.uk/globalassets/sitedocuments/standards-of-proficiency/nursing-associates/nursing-associates-proficiency-standards.pdf

SACKETT, D. L. *et al.*, 1996. Evidence based medicine: What it is and what it isn't [editorial]. *BMJ*, 312(7023), 71-72. https://doi.org/10.1136/bmj.312.7023.71

Part 2

Becoming and Being a Professional

4 Policies and legislation in health and social care practice

Ann Gorecki

Box 4.1: Contents

- Introduction
- What is legislation? Exploring key terms
- The legislative and policymaking process in the United Kingdom
- Key health and social care legislation: From 1946 to the present day
- Mental health legislation
- Learning disabilities legislation
- Children's services legislation
- Overarching legislation
- What next?

Box 4.2: Learning outcomes

By the end of this chapter, you should be able to

- Define key terms relating to policy and legislation
- Demonstrate knowledge of selected regulatory bodies
- Describe the legislation and policymaking process in the United Kingdom
- Articulate aspects of selected legislation
- Identify key concepts around the implementation of policy in health and social care practice.

Box 4.3: Keywords

- Legislation
- Bill
- Statutory guidance
- Non-statutory guidance
- Policymaking

DOI: 10.4324/9781003198338-6

- Code of practice
- Public sector regulatory body
- National Health Service
- Mental health
- Children's services
- Learning disabilities

Introduction

Legislation underpins all practice in health and social care (H&SC) and children's services, but its importance is not always recognised and understood by practitioners. This chapter aims to bridge this knowledge gap and explore how legislation translates into policy and how policy informs H&SC practice. We will examine the stages of the legislative and policymaking processes in the United Kingdom (UK). As we will see, much contemporary legislation is built upon previous laws, so this chapter presents a brief history of H&SC legislation from 1946 to the present day. We will then explore legislation specific to different areas of practice and discuss how public enquiries can change practice. Over-arching, more generic legislation that is central to effective patient-centred care will be discussed, and the implementation of policy in practice settings will also be considered.

What is legislation? exploring key terms

Activity 4.1: Can you define 'legislation'?

Before we explore definitions of 'legislation', can you define what this word means in one or two sentences?

Here are the definitions of some of the key terms used in this chapter:

- Legislation: a law or a set of laws passed by Parliament that have become an Act of Parliament
- Bill: a proposal either by the government (or, less commonly, by individual Members of Parliament) to introduce new legislation
- Statutory guidance: this explains what must be done to comply with the law
- Non-statutory guidance: this is a piece of legislation that is usually shorter and more accessible than statutory guidance and focuses on how to put the legislation into practice. The key difference from statutory guidance is that it is not enforceable by law
- Policy: The word 'policy' sometimes refers to government policy relating to broad principles (for example, the government's economic policy), but for the purpose of this chapter, 'policy' will refer to how specific courses of action are outlined within organisations. For example, there may be a policy within your organisation that are you are required to have a hepatitis B vaccination as part of your terms and conditions of employment

- Codes of practice: this relates to your occupational area as set out by the public sector regulatory body (see Panel 4.1) that oversees your profession. The code of practice constitutes the expected standards for that profession and provides key principles you should follow. You are accountable for your actions to the public sector regulatory body and, if you don't adhere to the relevant code, then you may be referred to the regulatory body as someone who is unfit to practise.

Activity 4.2: Identify a code of practice

Some codes of practice relate to practitioners for the United Kingdom, and some are specific to countries that are part of the United Kingdom. Look at the standards for your practice (and geographical) area and find at least one relevant standard that relates to communicating with service users and carers. Can you think of a recent example when you put it into practice?

Panel 4.1: Health and social care public sector regulatory bodies

Nursing associates, nurses and midwives are accountable to the Nursing and Midwifery Council (NMC) and are required to adhere to the NMC Code (2018) (www.nmc.org.uk/standards/code/) (UK-wide)

Allied health professionals are accountable to the Health and Care Professions Council and are required to adhere to their standards of conduct, performance and ethics (www.hcpc-uk.org/standards/standards-of-conduct-performance-and-ethics/) (UK-wide)

Social workers in England are accountable to Social Work England and are required to adhere to its code of standards (www.socialworkengland.org.uk/standards/professional-standards). Social workers in Wales are accountable to Social Care Wales (https://socialcare.wales/dealing-with-concerns/codes-of-practice-and-guidance). Those in Scotland are accountable to The Scottish Social Services Council (www.sssc.uk.com/the-scottish-social-services-council/sssc-codes-of-practice/) and Northern Irish social workers must abide by the code of practice of the Northern Ireland Social Care Council (https://niscc.info/app/uploads/2020/10/Standards-for-Social-Workers.pdf).

The legislative and policymaking process in the United Kingdom

To gain a better understanding of the process of developing legislation in the UK, we will now examine how laws are passed.

A bill can be introduced either in the House of Commons or in the House of Lords but needs to go through both Houses. See Panel 4.2 for an overview of the process of introducing a bill that starts in the House of Commons.

Panel 4.2: The process of creating legislation

- First reading: This is the first stage of a bill. There is no vote, and the bill is not discussed or amended
- Second reading: This is the stage when a bill is first debated. If the bill is defeated at this stage, then it can't be re-introduced in the same session
- Committee stage: This is the stage where deep scrutiny of a bill occurs
- Report (consideration) stage: This is the stage where Members of Parliament propose amendments to the bill
- Third reading: This is the final opportunity to debate a bill
- House of Lords: House of Lords follow the same stages as those followed in the House of Commons (although there are some differences). If a House of Commons bill is defeated in the House of Lords, then it does not go further in this process
- Consideration of amendments: After the House of Lords has considered a bill, it's sent back to the House of Commons or vice versa. If the House of Lords does not amend the bill, then it goes for royal assent
- Royal assent: This is the final stage of a bill where it goes to the monarch who agrees to make the bill an Act of Parliament

Institute for Government (2023).

The time taken for a bill to become an Act of Parliament varies, and as shown in Panel 4.2, the bill must pass through different stages. It can take several years for this process to be completed, especially when it is for a complex Act of Parliament. However, emergency measures—for example, some of those put into place during the COVID-19 pandemic—can be enacted much more quickly if needed.

We will now consider specific examples of H&SC legislation. These date back many decades. We begin our examination in 1946 and the founding of the National Health Service (NHS).

Key health and social care legislation: from 1946 to the present day

Creation of the National Health Service

One of the most important acts of legislation in the history of H&SC is the *NHS Act 1946*. This applied to England and Wales and provided the legislative basis for the founding of the NHS. In Scotland, the *NHS (Scotland) Act 1947* created the Department of Health for Scotland and the Scottish NHS. In Northern Ireland, the *Health Services Act (Northern Ireland) 1948* did the same. In all nations of the UK, the NHS came into effect on 5 July 1948.

Before the inception of the NHS, health services across the UK were fragmented and provided by charities, local authorities and private organisations. This meant that the healthcare a citizen received depended on where they lived and their ability to pay (Rivett 2020, 2022).

Many factors and events preceded, and contributed to, the founding of the NHS in 1948. These included

- The introduction of the wartime emergency medical service in 1939, which provided free hospital care for civilian air raid casualties. The Ministry of Health considered transitioning this successful initiative into a comprehensive, free and available one to all health services from 1943 onwards (Ministry of Health 1943, cited in Rivett 2022)
- The publication of *Beveridge Report* in 1942. This publication had identified the need for a 'cradle to grave' social programme and one of its proposals was a free, national health service (UK Parliament 1942)
- The voting into power of Clement Attlee's Labour party in 1945 with one of the largest majorities in history. As a socialist government, it was committed to a programme of nationalisation (putting private companies into public ownership), and this included introducing a national health service. Aneurin Bevan, Minister of Health, pushed for an even more radical reform, which meant nationalising municipal and voluntary hospitals

Under the 1946 Act, funding for this new health service had to come from income tax, with higher earners paying more tax but all users of the NHS receiving the same level of service. Fragmented and unequal healthcare service provision was replaced by universal and free-at-point-of-use access. NHS services were available according to patient need rather than the ability to pay. (Some previously free NHS services were withdrawn in the 1950s, notably prescriptions, dental work and provision of glasses. However, overall, the NHS remains free at the point of access. While legislation relating to some parts of the NHS—particularly its administration—has been amended since its inception, its main principles remain).

This new, comprehensive health service was designed to improve the physical and mental health of the people of England and Wales, prevent, diagnose and treat illness and provide or secure the effective provision of services.

Health and Social Care Act (2012)

More recent legislation to modernise the NHS was introduced with the *Health and Social Care Act (2012)*, which came into force on 1 April 2013 (UK Government 2012).

The Act was introduced by the government in response to both global and national concerns. As a result of austerity—and following the global financial crisis in 2008—the coalition government decided that some aspects of the NHS could be modernised and rationalised to stem increasing patient demand, curtail treatment costs and improve outcomes for patients.

The government claimed that the *Health and Social Care Act* showed 'commitment to put the public's health centre stage' (NHS Future Forum Report 2011 cited in Department of Health and Social Care 2012) and recognised the existence of major health inequalities in the UK. At a national level, a new agency—Public Health England—was created to bring together different organisations into one to improve accountability to the central government for national threats to health. At the same time, public health responsibilities were returned to local authorities (they were previously the responsibility of the now-defunct primary care Trusts [PCTs]). Local authorities were regarded as well placed to understand the impact of the social or wider determinants of health (for example, housing and economic development) on health issues.

Legislative changes aimed at improving patient outcomes included the introduction of a code of conduct for healthcare support workers, the recommendation to standardise induction processes for these workers and the creation of a voluntary register of healthcare support workers. The induction standards element was realised in the creation of the *Care Certificate* by *Health Education England*, *Skills for Health* and *Skills for Care* (Skills for Care 2022) introduced in 2015. This required all new healthcare support workers to complete the certificate within 12 weeks of starting their employment. However, the voluntary register of healthcare support workers was never introduced. It should also be noted that, although the certificate featured in the 2012 Act, the *Cavendish Review* (Cavendish 2013) was instrumental in pursuing its implementation (see Panel 4.3).

Panel 4.3: Policy into practice

Significant changes in practice can be prompted by public inquiries, often because of serious care failings. Reports about poor standards of care and a higher-than-average mortality rate were received at *Mid Staffordshire NHS Trust* (later *NHS Foundation Trust*) from 2005 to 2008. In 2009, Robert Francis QC began hearing evidence from patients and families who reported unacceptable care including patients left in soiled sheets or being unable to access food and drink. Francis published his inquiry report in 2010.

This was followed by a public inquiry in 2010. The final *Francis Report* was published in 2013 with 290 recommendations to try to ensure that such failures of care did not happen again. Recommendations included

- Ensuring the patient is at the centre of their care
- Openness and candour throughout the healthcare system
- Training and education for nurses should include good patient care
- Healthcare assistants should be registered and agree to work to a set of standards
- Every person should be responsible for their actions

Following the *Francis Report*, the *Cavendish Review* (2013) was commissioned to address the recommendation about registration for healthcare assistants and review healthcare assistants and support workers in the NHS and social care settings.

Camilla Cavendish found that healthcare assistants made up a third of the caring workforce and spent more time with patients than nurses. They should be seen as a 'critical strategic resource', yet many felt undervalued and overlooked (Cavendish 2013, p.5).

One of the recommendations was that a *Certificate of Fundamental Care* should be developed and introduced for all care workers and a *Higher Certificate of Fundamental Care* linked to more advanced competencies should be introduced.

These ideas were developed further by the *Shape of Caring Review* (Willis 2015), which recommended including people who use services in all aspects of a learner's journey, valuing the care assistant role and introducing career progression for healthcare assistants.

A direct response was the development of the role of a nursing associate. The underpinning qualification agreed was an H&SC foundation degree, and this also enabled further development of more specialist healthcare assistant practitioners (for example, therapy assistants). There is now a recognised career pathway for healthcare assistants and support workers, which some of you may be following.

Another result of these inquiries and reviews was the introduction of a *Care Certificate* as an induction tool for new employees and a development tool for existing healthcare assistants as a basic qualification to enable the improvement of practice (Francis 2013).

Under the 2012 Act, strategic health authorities and PCTs were abolished, and the responsibility of NHS commissioning was passed to NHS England at a national level and clinical commissioning groups (CCGs) at a local level. This represented a change in the control of the services commissioned by NHS England.

Activity 4.3: Read these additional resources (general)

As this chapter briefly addresses selected key legislation, look at resources that provide more information about your area of practice.

Health: Nuffield Trust–*NHS reform timeline* at: www.nuffieldtrust.org.uk/health-and-social-care-explained/nhs-reform-timeline

Social Care: Social Care Institute for Excellence (SCIE)'s *Key policy and legislation. A timeline of examples 1968–2008* at: www.scie.org.uk/assets/elearning/ipiac/ipiac01/resource/text/content/keyPolicy/keyPolicy.htm

See also Whittington *et al.* (2009).

The next section will provide an overview of the development of important legislation relating to different H&SC areas, focusing on one or two key pieces of legislation for each area. The areas are

- Mental health
- Learning disability
- Children's services

Some legislation considered in this section will be relevant to more than one practice area and other legislation applies to the general population but is of particular importance for H&SC practitioners.

Mental health legislation

Even if you are working in a general H&SC setting, it is likely that you will be supporting people living with mental health conditions. It is important, therefore, to know about the legislation underpinning the rights of people with mental health conditions.

The *Mental Health Act (1983)* is the main piece of legislation that covers a person's assessment, treatment and rights in England and Wales (UK Government 1983). (In Scotland, the Scottish Parliament has powers over mental health legislation and, in 2003, passed its own mental health act [*the Mental Health (Care and Treatment) (Scotland) Act 2003*], which came into effect in 2005.)

A person experiencing an acute mental health episode can be assessed and/or admitted for treatment on a voluntary basis. However, they may need to be detained under the *Mental Health Act* if they are deemed at risk of harm to themselves or others. This is often called 'being sectioned' and relates to a section of the Act. The following are some of the more commonly used sections of the act:

- *Section 135 of the Mental Health Act (1983)*: this section allows the police to enter a person's home and take them to a safe place so that a mental health assessment can be done. A warrant is required, and an application for a warrant must be made by an approved mental health professional (AMHP), where there is reasonable cause to believe that the person has a mental disorder and is being ill-treated or neglected; or is unable to look after themselves
- *Section 136*: this section applies to situations in a public place and allows the police to take a person to (or keep them at) a safe place. They can do this without a warrant if the person appears to have a mental disorder AND is in any place other than a house, flat or room where a person is living AND is in need of immediate 'care and control' (meaning the police may think it is necessary to keep the person or others safe). Before applying *section 136*, the police must consult a registered medical practitioner, a registered nurse or an AMHP occupational therapist or para-medic (MIND 2020)
- *Section 2, Admission for assessment*: when healthcare professionals as a team assess a person's mental health, they may decide that the best way to provide the care and treatment needed is to admit the person to a hospital and, unless he or she agrees to undergo voluntary treatment, they are placed under *section 2* for assessment. The team of professionals needed to enact *section 2* would include an AMHP and two doctors, one of whom is *section 12* approved, and one of whom is a registered practitioner, usually a doctor who is known to the person, such as their general practitioner (GP). The person can be kept in the hospital for up to 28 days

The mental health professional in charge of care and treatment under the MHA is known as the 'Responsible Clinician' or 'RC', and they can discharge the person from the section at any time if there is no longer a requirement for them to be sectioned.

If the RC decides that there is a need to continue treatment for longer than 28 days, then the person may be kept in the hospital under *section 3*. This enables a person to be kept in hospital for up to 6 months so that they can receive the treatment they require. Although consent is always sought, medication can be administered to the person with or without their consent. As with *section 2*, there will be an RC who is in charge of the person's care. If they consider that treatment needs to be extended beyond 6 months, then *section 3* can be continued for a further 6-month period and then for up to a year at a time (Rethink 2021; UK Government 1983).

Mental Capacity Act (2005)

The primary purpose of the *Mental Capacity Act (MCA) (2005)* was to promote and safeguard decision-making within a legal framework. It aims to do this by empowering people to make decisions for themselves where possible and protecting people who lack capacity by putting them in the centre of the decision-making process. It also aims to allow people to plan for a time in the future when they might lack capacity (Social Care Institute for Excellence 2021; UK Government 2005)

Mental capacity is assessed when a decision needs to be made. The *MCA* stipulates that a person is unable to make a decision if they cannot understand and retain information relevant to the decision or use that information as part of the process of decision-making or to communicate their decision. If the person is deemed to lack capacity, then any decision made for the person must be made in their best interests.

There are five principles of the *MCA*, which are as follows:

1. Presumption of a person's capacity: every adult has the right to make his or her own decisions and they must be assumed to have capacity to do so unless it is proven otherwise. This means that professionals cannot assume that someone cannot decide for themselves just because they have a particular medical condition or disability
2. Supporting a person to make decisions: a person must be given all practicable help before anyone treats them as not able to make their own decisions. This could mean finding an alternative way of communicating with the person
3. Unwise decisions: people have the right to make decisions that others might regard as unwise. Everyone has their own values, beliefs and preferences that may not be the same as those of other people
4. Best interests: anything done for or on behalf of a person who lacks mental capacity must be done in their best interests
5. Less restrictive option: someone making a decision for a person who lacks capacity must consider whether it is possible to decide or act in a way that would interfere less with the person's rights and freedoms of action, or whether there is a need to decide or act at all (Social Care Institute for Excellence 2021).

Mental Health Act (2007)

The *Mental Health Act (2007)* amended the *Mental Health Act (1983)*. It simplified the original Act's definition of a mental disorder to 'any disorder or disability of the mind'. Significantly, by extending the definition of 'mental disorder', this Act included other conditions such as dementia, changes in behaviour due to brain injury, mental disorders due to drug use and autistic spectrum disorders.

To safeguard children, it introduced a new requirement for children and young people under the age of 18 years to be treated in age-appropriate settings. This followed concerns about children being detained on adult wards and the possibility of this having a negative impact on their recovery.

The *Mental Health Act 2007* also introduced some changes to the *MCA*. The changes were prompted following a situation when a person with autism who was a voluntary patient continued to be detained as the hospital claimed that the decision was made in their best interests. This was challenged by their family, and it became known as the 'Bournewood gap'. To close the gap, the *Mental Health Act 2007* amended the *MCA*

2005 and introduced *Deprivation of Liberty Safeguards*. This meant that, before anyone could be deprived of their liberty (either by restraint or by restrictions to their liberty), authorisation must be obtained from the local authority (UK Government 2007; King's Fund 2008).

Learning disabilities legislation

Most legislation relating to people with learning disabilities now—rightly—focuses on promoting and upholding their rights. Historically, this was not always the case and, although general H&SC legislation (such as the *NHS Act (1948)*) implicitly includes people with learning disabilities, the system has often excluded them and denied them basic rights.

This begins in childhood and outside of H&SC settings. Before 1970—when the *Education (Handicapped Children) Act* was passed—children with learning disabilities did not even have the right to education. With the passing of this Act, there was a growth in the building of special schools (UK Government 1970).

In 1970, the *Chronically Sick and Disabled Persons Act* was passed. This explicitly included people with learning disabilities and required local authorities to support people with practical assistance and recreational activities in the community. The reality was, however, that many people with learning disabilities were housed in long-term hospitals (UK Government 1970).

The challenge of people who fell between H&SC services (including people with learning disabilities) was highlighted by Griffiths (1988). In bringing this issue to the fore, and discussing the fact that people with learning disabilities were receiving inadequate support more generally, Griffiths' work is considered to have paved the way for the move from institutional care to community-based support.

Griffiths observed that the lack of success and development of community care up to this point was down to the lack of leadership and responsibility, describing community care as 'everybody's distant cousin but nobody's baby'.

Other legislation of interest here includes the 2001 White Paper *Valuing People* (Department of Health 2001). It should also be noted that the *MCA 2005* is discussed in the mental health section of this chapter, but it is important to mention here that it acknowledged that people with learning disabilities have the right to make their own decisions about their care if they have the capacity to do so.

The *2009 Autism Act* was the first piece of legislation specific to a learning disability and ensured statutory provision for adults with an autism spectrum condition. It committed the government to publish an adult autism strategy to transform services, and the strategy was published in 2010 with further statutory guidance for local authorities and the NHS published in 2015 (UK Government 2009; Department of Health 2015).

The *Care Act 2014* specified that local authorities must carry out an assessment of anyone who appears to require care and support, regardless of their likely eligibility for state-funded care. There was also a focus on the assessment of the person's needs and how they impact on their well-being, and the outcomes they want to achieve. This was also significant for people with learning disabilities, as it specified the need to recognise their agency (Social Care Institute for Excellence 2016; UK Government 2014).

Poor outcomes for people with learning disabilities are significant. The 2020 annual report from the Learning Disabilities Mortality Review programme (cited in NICE 2021) showed that the average age at death for people with a learning disability is 23 years younger for men and 27 years younger for women than that of the wider population. It further found that 41% of adult deaths were due to treatable medical causes and 24% were due to preventable medical causes. Most of the avoidable deaths in people with a learning disability were because timely and effective treatment was not given (NICE 2021). Although the reasons are multi-factorial, barriers in communication and gaps in the understanding of the needs of people with a learning disability can indicate difficulty in obtaining treatment for health conditions.

Activity 4.4: Read these additional resources (learning disabilities)

As this chapter briefly addresses selected legislation, look at this resource that provides more detail about learning disabilities.

   Open University–*Timeline of learning disability history* at www.open.ac.uk/health-and-social-care/research/shld/timeline-learning-disability-history.

Children's services legislation

The main emphasis of the legislation we will now consider relates to the safeguarding of children and young people and how it aims to protect them from abuse. Current legislation and guidelines reflect the fact that safeguarding children is everyone's responsibility so, even if your job role does not involve working directly with children, it is still important for you to be able to play your part in safeguarding children.

   The key piece of legislation for safeguarding children and young people is the *Children Act (1989)* (UK Government 1989). The main principles of the Act are:

- The welfare of the child is paramount
- Professionals must work together in partnership
- Parents have responsibilities for their children, not absolute rights
- Children should preferably be raised within their own family

The law also established two levels of areas of concern:

- Children and young people can be deemed to be 'in need' when extra support is required
- Serious concerns raise the possibility that they are at risk of 'serious harm' if parents or carers fail to ensure the child can be safe and thrive
  (*Children Act (1989)*, cited in Lindon and Webb 2016)

The *Children Act (2004)* built on, but did not replace, the *Children Act (1989)*. The amendments were deemed necessary following the *Laming Inquiry* (Laming 2003) into the murder of Victoria Climbié. Many recommendations made by Laming were related to increasing and improving communication between professionals and inter-agency working. Following the publication of Every Child Matters, (UK Government 2003) a national role of Children's Commissioner was created, and Local Safeguarding Children's Boards were established by local authorities to co-ordinate and ensure the effectiveness of professionals and organisations with a responsibility to safeguard children.

Working Together to Safeguard Children (Department for Education 2018) is statutory guidance on how professionals should work together to safeguard and promote the welfare of children. By emphasising the need for effective inter-agency working, it established the premise that safeguarding is the responsibility of anyone who encounters children and families (and not just certain professionals).

If you ever have concerns about a child or young person as part of your professional role, then you should report any concerns—however minor—to your line manager or the Safeguarding Lead in your organisation. If you have concerns outside of your role, please see Panel 4.4 below.

Panel 4.4: Links to National Society for the Prevention of Cruelty to Children

Links to the National Society for the Prevention of Cruelty to Children guidelines on recognising signs of child abuse and what to do if you suspect that a child is being abused can be accessed here: www.nspcc.org.uk/what-is-child-abuse/spotting-signs-child-abuse/ and www.nspcc.org.uk/keeping-children-safe/reporting-abuse/.

Activity 4.5: Additional resources (children and young people)

As this chapter briefly addresses selected legislation only on children and young people, take a look at resources that provide more information l related to your area of practice.

Children's Services: National Society for the Protection of Children (NSPCC)– *History of safeguarding children in the UK* at https://learning.nspcc.org.uk/child-protection-system/history-of-child-protection-in-the-uk.

Overarching legislation

Many pieces of legislation applying to all occupational areas are particularly relevant to H&SC practitioners. These include:

- *Data Protection Act 2018* (UK Government 2018): This Act relates to the way that information is stored and handled and the need for maintaining confidentiality. Its importance is emphasised in professional codes of practice and within Trust and other organisations' policies, which you should make yourself aware of
- *Health and Safety at Work Act 1974* (UK Government 1974): This Act defines the responsibilities of your employer to maintain a healthy and safe working environment and your rights in this regard. Although the primary responsibility lies with the employer, workers have a duty to take care of their own health and safety and that of others and to report issues of concern. This is important in H&SC settings, as there are many factors that can compromise the working environment. For example, the Act specifies the need to provide sufficient personal protective equipment to ensure adequate protection from infection and the requirement for safe staffing levels to be maintained

- The *Reporting of Injuries, Diseases and Dangerous Occurrences Regulations (RIDDOR) 2013* (Health and Safety Executive, 2013): This focuses on the requirement to report any accidents and 'near misses' that occur in the workplace to ensure lessons are learned and future accidents prevented
- *Control of Substances Hazardous to Health Regulations (COSHH) 2002* (Health and Safety Executive, 2002): This regulation places the responsibility with the employer for safe storage and control of substances deemed hazardous to health. An example of a substance is oxygen, which, whilst not generally hazardous in itself, poses a potential fire risk and its use needs to be controlled.
- The *Equality Act 2010* (UK Government 2010): This Act brought together several pieces of anti-discriminatory legislation by defining protected characteristics Examples of how it is particularly relevant in H&SC include
- Ensuring people receiving care and the workers providing care are protected from being treated unfairly because of protected characteristics
- The need for public organisations including NHS Trusts to have due regard to the need to eliminate unlawful discrimination, harassment and victimisation
- Hospitals, care homes and GP surgeries ensuring they remove barriers to access by making reasonable adjustments (Social Care Institute for Excellence 2020)

Your organisation or Trust policies will be underpinned by these pieces of legislation, and there is often a requirement to complete training in these areas to ensure understanding and compliance.

What next?

As we have seen throughout the chapter, legislation does not remain static and new Acts build on and develop earlier legislation. At the time of writing this chapter, several pieces of legislation have been passed or are nearing completion.

Health and Care Act (2022)

The most recent piece of specific legislation that has passed into law is the *Health and Care Act 2022* (UK Government 2022a). As the first major NHS reform in 10 years, it is a significant piece of legislation. Building on proposals for change set out by NHS England in their *Long-Term Plan*, it will increase partnership arrangements between the NHS and Local Authority care provision.

Integrated care systems (which have been in place informally in recent years) have been formalised by the Act and will replace Clinical Commissioning Groups. These systems should enable communication and co-operation between health organisations, with social care to be simplified.

It also grants the Secretary of Health authority over the health service and expands their powers. Examples of these powers are the potential to create new NHS Trusts or to intervene in local service restructuring. Timmins (2021), considering these proposals before the law was passed, argued against that this development is unwieldly, necessitating ministers' involvement in 'every decision about every service change'. He also argues that the new powers of direction over NHS England forms a dangerous precedent for introducing major changes without debate.

For people with learning disabilities, the *Health and Care Act 2022* will enshrine mandatory training for all H&SC staff on learning disabilities and autism. The *Down Syndrome Act 2022* (UK Government 2022b) was passed in April 2022 with the aim to make provision to meet the needs of people with Down Syndrome.

Mental Health Act

Following recommendations of a review by Professor Sir Simon Wessley in 2018, there is a mental health bill currently going through the legislative process to overhaul the *Mental Health Act 1983* (UK Government 1983). It is proposed that it will limit the extent to which the Act can be used to detain people with autism and people with learning disabilities and will compel practitioners to ensure more consideration is given to treatment preferences if patients are detained under the Act. It also aims to address the disparity of numbers of people from black and minority ethnic groups and unequal treatment for those who are detained under the Act (Wessley 2018).

Summary

This chapter examined selected examples of H&SC policy and legislation from 1946 to the present day. It also discussed the political context of policymaking and considered the origins of some legislation in scandals in care settings such as the Mid Staffordshire NHS Trust one. Legislation related to mental health, learning disability and children's services was discussed, and upcoming policy developments were explored. All H&SC practitioners need to be familiar with the relevant legislation, understand codes of practice in their area and stay updated about developments in their care setting.

Box 4.4: Key learning points

- Legislation refers to a law or a set of laws passed by Parliament and that have become an Act of Parliament
- Legislation and codes of practice underpin all areas of health and social care practice
- The National Health Service came into effect in 1948 following the *NHS Act 1946*
- The *Health and Social Care Act (2012)* led to a major re-organisation of the NHS
- Safeguarding children is everyone's responsibility even if your job role does not involve working directly with children
- Health and social care practitioners have an important role in putting legislation into practice and upholding the rights of themselves and their patients.

References

CAVENDISH, C., 2013. *The Cavendish Review: An independent review into healthcare assistants and support workers in the NHS and social care settings*. London: The Stationery Office.
DEPARTMENT FOR EDUCATION, 2018. *Working together to safeguard children*. London: The Stationery Office.

DEPARTMENT OF HEALTH, 2012. *Transforming care: A national response to Winterbourne View Hospital: Department of Health Review final report*. London: The Stationery Office.

DEPARTMENT OF HEALTH, 2015. *Adult autism strategy*. London: The Stationery Office.

DEPARTMENT OF HEALTH AND SOCIAL CARE, 2012. *New focus for public health fact sheet* [viewed 17 August 2022]. Available from: www.gov.uk/government/publications/health-and-soc ial-care-act-2012-fact-sheets

DEPARTMENT OF HEALTH, 2001. *Valuing people*. London: The Stationery Office.

FRANCIS, R., 2013. *Report of the Mid Staffordshire NHS Foundation Trust public inquiry*. London: HMSO.

GRIFFITHS, R., 1988. *Community care: Agenda for action. London* HMSO.

HEALTH AND SAFETY EXECUTIVE, 2002. *Control of substances hazardous to health regulations* (COSHH) [viewed 17 August 2022]. Available from: www.hse.gov.uk/coshh/

HEALTH AND SAFETY EXECUTIVE, 2013. *Reporting of injuries, diseases and dangerous occurrences regulations 2013* [viewed 17 August 2022]. Available from: www.hse.gov.uk/riddor/

INSTITUTE FOR GOVERNMENT, 2023. *The legislative process in parliament* [viewed 20 January 2023]. Available from: www.instituteforgovernment.org.uk/article/explainer/legislative-process-parliament

KING'S FUND, 2008. *Briefing: Mental Health Act 2007* [viewed 17 August 2022]. Available from: www.kingsfund.org.uk/sites/default/files/briefing-mental-health-act-2007-simon-lawton-smith-kings-fund-december-2008.pdf

LAMING, L., 2003. *The Victoria Climbié Inquiry*. London: HMSO.

LINDON, J. and J. WEBB, 2016. *Safeguarding and child protection*. 5th ed. London: Hodder Education.

MIND, 2020. *Sectioning* [viewed 17 August 2022]. Available from: www.mind.org.uk/informat ion-support/legal-rights/sectioning/overview/

NICE, 2021. *NICE impact people with a learning disability* [viewed 10 July 2023]. Available from: https://www.nice.org.uk/about/what-we-do/into-practice/measuring-the-use-of-nice-guidance/impact-of-our-guidance/nice-impact-people-with-a-learning-disability

RETHINK, 2021. *Rights and restrictions* [viewed 17 August 2022]. Available from: www.rethink.org/Factsheets/9920/Mental%20Health%20Act%201983%20factsheet

RIVETT, G., 2020. *The development of the London hospital system 1823–2020*. 2nd ed. London: King's Fund.

RIVETT, G., 2022. *The history of the NHS* [viewed 17 August 2022]. Available from: www.nuffie ldtrust.org.uk/health-and-social-care-explained/the-history-of-the-nhs

SKILLS FOR CARE, 2022. *Developing your workforce: Care Certificate*. Leeds: Skills for Care.

SOCIAL CARE INSTITUTE FOR EXCELLENCE, 2016. *The Care Act 2014* [viewed 17 August 2022]. Available from: www.scie.org.uk/care-act-2014/assessment-and-eligibility/

SOCIAL CARE INSTITUTE FOR EXCELLENCE, 2020. *Equality Act 2010* [viewed 17 August 2022]. Available from: www.scie.org.uk/key-social-care-legislation/equality-act

SOCIAL CARE INSTITUTE FOR EXCELLENCE, 2021. *Mental Capacity Act at a glance* [viewed 17 August 2022]. Available from: www.scie.org.uk/mca/introduction/mental-capacity-act-2005-at-a-glance

TIMMINS, N., 2021. *The ministerial powers proposed in the Health and Care Bill should not be granted* [viewed 17 August 2022]. *Institute for Government [blog]*. Available from: www.institu teforgovernment.org.uk/blog/ministerial-powers-health-care-bill

UK GOVERNMENT, 1970. *Education (Handicapped Children Act 1970)* [viewed 17 August 2022]. Available from: www.legislation.gov.uk/ukpga/1970/52/contents/enacted

UK GOVERNMENT, 1974. *Health and Safety at Work Act 1974* [viewed 17 August 2022]. Available from: www.legislation.gov.uk/ukpga/1974/37/contents

UK GOVERNMENT, 1983. *Mental Health Act 1983* [viewed 17 August 2022]. Available from: www.legislation.gov.uk/ukpga/1983/20/contents

UK GOVERNMENT, 1989. *Children Act 1989* [viewed 17 August 2022]. Available from: www.legislation.gov.uk/ukpga/1989/41/contents

UK GOVERNMENT, 2003. *Every Child Matters 2003* [viewed 17 August 2022]. Available from: https://assets.publishing.service.gov.uk/government/uploads/system/uploads/attachment_data/file/272064/5860.pdf

UK GOVERNMENT, 2005. *Mental Capacity Act 2005* [viewed 17 August 2022]. Available from: www.legislation.gov.uk/ukpga/2005/9/contents

UK GOVERNMENT, 2007. *Mental Health Act 2007* [viewed 17 August 2022]. Available from: www.legislation.gov.uk/ukpga/2007/12/contents

UK GOVERNMENT, 2009. *Autism Act 2009* [viewed 17 August 2022]. Available from: www.legislation.gov.uk/ukpga/2009/15/contents

UK GOVERNMENT, 2010. *Equality Act 2010* [viewed 17 August 2022]. Available from: www.legislation.gov.uk/ukpga/2010/15/contents

UK GOVERNMENT, 2012. *The Health and Social Care Act 2012* [viewed 17 August 2022]. Available from: www.legislation.gov.uk/ukpga/2012/7/contents/enacted

UK GOVERNMENT, 2014. *Care Act* [viewed 17 August 2022]. Available from: www.legislation.gov.uk/ukpga/2014/23/contents/enacted

UK GOVERNMENT, 2018. *Data Protection Act 2018* [viewed 17 August 2022]. Available from: www.legislation.gov.uk/ukpga/2018/12/contents/enacted

UK GOVERNMENT, 2022a. *The Health and Social Care Act 2022* [viewed 17 August 2022]. Available from: www.legislation.gov.uk/uksi/2022/15/contents/made

UK GOVERNMENT, 2022b. *Down Syndrome Act 2022* [viewed 17 August 2022]. Available from: https://bills.parliament.uk/bills/2899

UK PARLIAMENT, 1942. *Social insurance and allied services, para 428*. Report by Sir William Beveridge. London: HMSO.

WESSLEY, S., 2018. *Modernising the Mental Health Act: Increasing choice, reducing compulsion*. London: Department of Health and Social Care.

WHITTINGTON, C. et al., 2009. *Key policy and legislation with implications for interprofessional and inter-agency collaboration (IPIAC): A timeline of examples 1968–2008*. London: Social Care Institute for Excellence (SCIE).

WILLIS, L., 2015. *Raising the bar: Shape of caring: A review of the future education and training of registered nurses and care assistants*. Leeds: HEE/NMC. (Lord Willis Independent Chair).

5 Becoming a health and social care professional

Mandy Lyons and Lisa Arai

Box 5.1: Contents

- Introduction
- What does 'professionalism' mean?
- Developing professional identity
- Becoming a professional: Key concepts
- Registration as a health and social care professional: New role and new responsibilities

---

Box 5.2: Learning outcomes

By the end of this chapter, you should be able to

- Reflect on what is meant by professional identity
- Discuss the importance of person-centred care
- Explain accountability, safeguarding and candour
- Discuss the importance of preceptorship
- Evaluate the key concepts of self-evaluation and reflection
- Identify strategies for looking after yourself
- Identify professional bodies and understand their processes for when things go wrong.

Box 5.3: Keywords

- Professional identity
- Practice
- Person-centred care

DOI: 10.4324/9781003198338-7

- Accountability
- Safeguarding
- Whistleblowing
- Self-evaluation
- Self-care
- Registration
- Preceptorship

Introduction

Everybody who works in a health and social care (H&SC) setting can rightly be considered a 'professional', even those without Nursing and Midwifery Council (NMC) or another type of registration. Regardless of what kind of practitioner you are—whether you are a newly qualified nursing associate, an experienced nurse or a mid-career healthcare assistant practitioner (HCAP)—you are required to be professional in all aspects of your work. Given this, this chapter explores what it means to be a professional within an H&SC setting and examines the concept of professional identity, the role of governing bodies, the importance of professional standards and the paramountcy of accountability. Safeguarding and protection of the public will be discussed, as will the need for reflection on practice and the importance of career development. The supporting activities will enable you to explore these concepts in more detail and consider their application to your specific role and area of practice.

This chapter is aimed especially at current or future practitioners, but readers not currently in practice, or those who are not planning to work in an H&SC setting in the near or more distant future, will benefit from learning about key concepts relevant to practice such as accountability, whistleblowing or safeguarding. While reading this chapter and engaging with activities, bear in mind that 'becoming' a professional never stops; it is an ongoing process.

What does 'professionalism' mean?

Activity 5.1: What do you think 'professionalism' means?

Before we explore what it means to become a professional, what do you think 'professionalism' means? Make a note of your thoughts.

What does it mean to be a 'professional'?

Did you identify key words associated with being a professional, such as 'trust', 'expertise', 'standards', 'reliability', 'integrity', 'respect', 'ethical', 'honesty', 'competence', 'accountability', 'commitment' and 'self-awareness'?

There is a large body of scholarly commentary on being a professional, the attributes of a professional and professionalism more broadly. Caza and Creary (2016) note that, in previous eras, an individual would be considered a professional only after they had completed the education and training necessary to enter a profession *and* after they had internalised the values and norms associated with that profession. Now, they observe, membership of a profession is based solely on attainment of skills or education, and the term 'professional' tends to be used as an adjective rather than a noun (so that it's about *how* individuals carry out their work rather than the nature of their work). Exactly what it means to be a professional appears to be widely contested within this literature (Brotherton and Parker 2013).

The essence of being a professional is to demonstrate integrity and commitment to delivering a high standard of public service. It is expected that any professional will have undergone education and training to achieve a standard of proficiency and expertise to enable them to do this.

It has been suggested that to really be classed as a professional requires membership of a professional regulatory body because this indicates that the professional has accepted that they will be held accountable for their actions and behaviours (Balthazard 2015). However, this is a contentious point and one you may wish to explore when considering professional identity; for example, this would define a nursing associate as a professional, as they are registered with the NMC but not the HCAP who currently does not require registration from the Health and Care Professions Council (HCPC) yet has undergone further education similar to the nursing associate in achieving a foundation degree in H&SC.

The term 'professional' can be applied to many types of behaviours or attributes—we talk about 'professional behaviour', for example, or 'professional values' and a 'professional identity'.

Developing professional identity

Activity 5.2: What is professional identity?

What is professional identity? Take 5 minutes to write in your own words what you think is meant by this term?

When considering professional identity, did you consider how others perceive you and your role, including peers, other professionals, members of the public and service users?

'Professional identity' as a term is not commonly used in practice and appears to be a confusing, often misunderstood concept within H&SC. Much of the existing literature exploring professional identity focusses on organisational identity and employer expectation of different roles. Nursing has a history of struggling to establish its identity and distance itself from the long-standing image of being subordinate to the medical profession (Ten Hoeve, Jansen and Roodbol 2014).

Caza and Creary (2016) write that: 'A professional identity is an individual's image of who they are as a professional ... the constellation of attributes, beliefs, values, motives and experiences that people use to define themselves in their professional capacity' (p.4).

Neary (2014) says that: 'Professional identity is the concept which describes how we perceive ourselves within our occupational context and how we communicate this to others' (p.14).

To establish a professional identity, individuals should first consider the following:

- How they perceive themselves
- How do they believe others perceive them and their role?
- What are employer expectations of their role?
- How do the wider public perceive their role? Does this vary depending on the country they are working in and how gender is viewed in that society?
- How does professional identity affect interprofessional teamworking?
- What are the barriers to establishing a positive professional identity?

It has been argued that the foundation of the professional identity of an individual or groups (such as nurses and physiotherapists) comes from their perception of how they are viewed by society; if they assume that society holds them in high regard and their public image is positive, then this boosts self-concept, and vice versa (Ten Hoeve, Jansen and Roodbol 2014).

Importance of being a professional

Being a professional and having a professional identity has many advantages. These include:

- Giving meaning to work and to life
- Shaping attitudes to work (this, in turn, can impact the care of patients, clients and service users)
- Helping individuals to progress in their careers
- Promoting networking with, and support from, others (especially where individuals have joined professional organisations)

Following the publication of Francis Report (Francis 2013) exploring the scandal of widespread negligence and sub-standard patient care within Mid Staffordshire National Health Service (NHS) Foundation Trust (see also chapters 4 and 11), there was a significant loss of public confidence in healthcare services and the nursing profession. When the NMC Code was later revised (in 2018) to include the new nursing associate role, a key aspect of nursing practice highlighted was the requirement for registrants to actively promote professionalism and trust to rebuild a positive public image of nursing.

More recently during the COVID-19 pandemic, the media portrayed healthcare services in a positive way (Bennett, James and Kelly 2020), thereby enhancing the public image of nursing and healthcare practitioners (this was despite unprecedented demands on care provision meaning changes in services and limited general access to healthcare).

Activity 5.3: Reflect on your professional identity

Take time to reflect on your professional identity throughout your career. As professional identity is dynamic, your perceptions may change depending on your stage of education and professional development.

Becoming a professional: key concepts

In this section, we will examine several concepts relevant to becoming an H&SC professional and developing professional identity. This is not an exhaustive examination, and you are encouraged to read around these concepts.

Person-centred care

Person-centred care has been widely discussed in relation to the care of older people, and particularly within dementia care and caring for people with learning disability (Ross, Tod and Clarke 2014), highlighting that when care is focused on the person's unique needs it has a positive effect, not only on the person receiving care but also on their family and the job satisfaction of nursing staff.

When the six 'Cs' in nursing care were first established by Jane Cummings, Chief Nursing Officer, in 2012, they were promoted as a set of values for all H&SC staff to embed in practice to support the delivery of high-quality, person-centred care (Cummings and Bennett 2012).

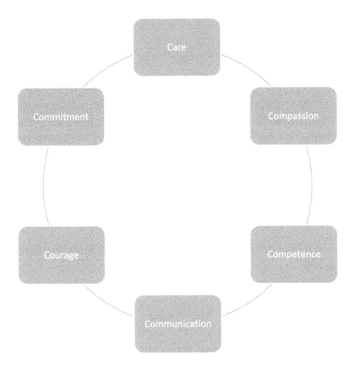

Figure 5.1 The six 'Cs' of nursing
Adapted from: Cummings and Bennett (2012)

Activity 5.4: Watch these videos on the six 'Cs' and person-centred care

Before moving on, you may find the following videos about the six 'Cs' and person-centred care helpful:

- www.youtube.com/watch?v=Z7t0Ce8uKTc
- www.nmc.org.uk/standards/code/code-in-action/person-centred-care

---

Some time ago, in his exploration of dementia care, Kitwood (1997) identified that effective implementation of person-centred care requires knowledgeable and enthusiastic staff working in teams that are open, respectful and trusting of one another. The importance of relationships and personal qualities of staff are essential to the delivery of person-centred care, but conflict between organisational and management priorities and what busy, front-line staff see as patient priorities can sometimes present challenges in the delivery of person-centred care (Ross, Tod and Clarke 2014). The key to delivering person-centred care is to ensure you value the unique qualities of each individual you care for, prioritising them, and ensuring you work with them to meet their individual holistic needs (Nursing and Midwifery Council 2018). See chapter 9 for a fuller discussion of person-centred care.

Accountability

This is a central concept in H&SC practice and is mentioned several times in the Nursing and Midwifery Council Code (2018) ('Be accountable for your decisions to delegate tasks and duties to other people'). Accountability is about helping practitioners to provide safe, high-quality, patient-centred care and ensuring they work within their competence and scope of practice. However, despite its importance, accountability may be difficult to define. A key word often associated with accountability is 'responsibility'.

Activity 5.5: Accountability and responsibility

Take a moment to reflect on what these two words mean to you. How do they differ? Jot down your thoughts.

You might have written some of the following for Activity 5.5:

- Being answerable for your actions
- Willingness to take responsibility for decisions
- Links to legal duties, policies and obligations (see also chapter 4)
- Readiness to accept the consequences of action
- Empowers clinical decision making
- Reduces opportunities for corruption, abuse of power and poor practice
- Supports the improvement of care for patients/service users

(Adapted from: Savage and Moore 2004).

Professional accountability supports H&SC practitioners to work within a safe framework of practice, but individuals may have a different understanding and interpretation of accountability. For some, accountability may be linked to blame, which risks defensive practice and resentment of management and authority (Caulfield 2005).

Accountability is closely linked to delegation, so you should ensure personal competency before accepting any delegated duty and ascertain the competency of others before you delegate any aspect of care to them. Failing to acknowledge deficits in knowledge and skills, and not accepting responsibility while also lacking insight can lead to poor, potentially unsafe patient-centred care (Peate 2019).

Working within professional role boundaries and a personal sphere of competency is essential to the delivery of safe, patient-centred care and must be considered during any delegation of care. Health Education England (2017) considers delegation to be: 'the handing over of specific tasks or areas of responsibility *while retaining accountability for those tasks/areas of work*', which demonstrates the intrinsic link between delegation and accountability (italicisation added).

The Health and Care Professions Council (2021) links accountability closely to safeguarding, consent and confidentiality; it stresses the importance of being able to justify your decisions and actions and your responsibility to raise concerns about care provision if required.

Activity 5.6: Look at these resources on accountability

The Nursing and Midwifery Council discusses accountability throughout its 2018 code of practice (Nursing and Midwifery Council 2018), and it has also published supplementary information on accountability and delegation, which can be accessed here: www.nmc.org.uk/globalassets/sitedocuments/nmc-publications/delegation-and-accountability-supplementary-information-to-the-nmc-code.pdf

The Royal College of Nursing's Principles of Delegation (2022) state that

- Delegation must always be in the best interest of the patient and not to save time or money
- The support worker must be suitably trained to perform the intervention
- Full records of training given should be kept
- Evidence that support workers' competence has been assessed should be recorded, preferably against recognised standards
- There should be clear guidelines and protocols in place so that the support worker is not required to make clinical judgements on their own
- The role should be within the support worker's job description
- The team and support staff need to be informed that the activity has been delegated
- The person who delegates the activity must ensure that an appropriate level of supervision is available and that the support worker has the opportunity for mentorship. The level of supervision and feedback needed depends on the knowledge and competence of the support worker, needs of the patient/client, service setting and activities assigned

- Support workers must have ongoing development to make sure their competency is maintained
- The whole process must be assessed to identify any risks

See www.rcn.org.uk/Professional-Development/Accountability-and-delegation/Accountability-and-delegation-case-studies for more information.

Panel 5.1: Accountability case study

If we follow the principle that any actions or omissions in our delivery of care are based on applying clinical judgement and making a decision, then accountability means that we must be able to explain and justify our decision-making processes and take responsibility for the outcome (Gallagher and Hodge 2012). Read the case study below and answer the questions that follow it to explore accountability in more detail.

Case study

A healthcare assistant (HCA) has recently joined your community-based, integrated care team. You met her during her initial induction period and are aware that she has several years' experience working in the endoscopy department at a local acute hospital trust. You have been asked by your line manager if the new staff member could shadow you during your morning visits to housebound individuals.

While visiting an elderly gentleman with dementia who requires a blood test for routine monitoring of his long-term conditions, your work phone rings just as you are explaining the purpose of your visit to the patient. As you excuse yourself to take the call outside, the HCA asks: 'Is it ok if I take this patient's blood? I've done phlebotomy for years so this is nice and straightforward for me and will save us time.' As you are very busy and believe the call is to add another visit to your already full list, you say 'yes'.

On return, the patient is clearly distressed and his wife is not happy that he had been left with someone he didn't know, and she is complaining that: 'This new nurse doesn't know what she is doing—she couldn't even find a vein and now she wants to have a third go. This is not good enough and I am going to 'phone to complain and insist that the lovely matron we met recently is the only one who comes to visit us in future!'

- What are your initial thoughts about the outcome of this episode of patient-centred care?
- Was a person-centred approach to care adopted?
- Was delegation in the best interests of the patient?
- Who holds accountability in this situation?

You can see possible responses to these questions in Panel 5.2.

Panel 5.2: Possible responses to the accountability case study

- *What are your initial thoughts about the outcome of this episode of patient care?*
  The patient with dementia was left feeling distressed and in discomfort due to failed phlebotomy attempts. The wife was very dissatisfied with the care her husband had received and felt 'let down' by the team that usually care for him, to the point of wanting to make a complaint.
- *Was a person-centred approach to care adopted?*
  Initially, you, as the lead H&SC professional, began to explain the purpose of the visit to the patient. However, you were distracted by a 'phone call and allowed the heavy workload for that day to influence your decision-making rather than focussing on the individual needs of the patient. You should have recognised that the patient did not know this new member of the team, which is especially significant in case of someone with dementia.
- *Was delegation in the best interests of the patient?*
  It would be difficult to justify a 'yes' response to this question considering the poor outcome. The patient did not know the new HCA and you didn't know the new HCA well and may not have checked whether or not she was competent in phlebotomy (and, even if she had gained proficiency in phlebotomy within the Endoscopy Suite, this was a new context of care in someone's home with a patient who may have anxiety due to dementia). It was not in the patient's best interest to leave the HCA unsupervised during this episode of care.
- *Who holds accountability in this situation?*

A number of professionals hold accountability. These are:

- The HCA herself, as she offered to take blood from a previously unknown patient (especially one with dementia), unsupervised, and she accepted the delegated task
- You, as the lead H&SC professional who delegated the clinical procedure (possibly without checking the HCA's proficiency) and then left her unsupervised with a vulnerable patient
- The registered nurse, for delegating the visit to a vulnerable patient with complex comorbidities in the first place to two unregistered professionals and for delegating supervision of the new HCA to another unregistered H&SC worker when she had joined the team only recently. The new HCA therefore had had little opportunity for supervised practice in this new clinical environment to confirm her proficiencies.

Safeguarding

All professionals in H&SC, and in other areas such as education, have safeguarding responsibilities. What does this mean? NHS England defines this as:

protecting a citizen's health, well-being and human rights; enabling them to live free from harm, abuse and neglect. It is an integral part of providing high-quality healthcare. Safeguarding children, young people and adults is a collective responsibility' (NHS England 2019).

People who need protection the most include children, young people and adults at risk (for example, disabled adults). Safeguarding is underpinned by policy and legislation (see chapter 4). In the NHS, staff members are required to adhere to the Safeguarding, Accountability and Assurance Framework (NHS England 2019).

Health providers are required under statute and regulation to have effective arrangements in place to safeguard and promote the welfare of children and adults at risk of harm and abuse in every service that they deliver. Providers must demonstrate that safeguarding is embedded at every level in their organisation with effective governance processes evident. Providers must assure themselves, the regulators, and their commissioners that safeguarding arrangements are robust and are in place.

Activity 5.7: Do you know the safeguarding processes in your workplace?

Take time to look up safeguarding policies in your workplace. Ensure you stay updated on mandatory safeguarding training.

Whistleblowing and raising concerns

Whistleblowers are workers who report wrong-doing in their workplaces in the name of the public interest. Whistleblowers are protected by law and should not suffer any hardship (such as loss of employment) if they disclose poor or illegal practice.

NHS England publishes the number of whistleblowing disclosures annually. During the period 1 April 2021 to 31 March 2022, 110 whistleblowing disclosures were made to NHS England relating to primary care organisations. Action was taken in 59% of the cases. In the same period, 96 whistleblowing disclosures were made relating to secondary care, and action was taken in 70% of the cases (NHS England 2022a).

Panel 5.3: Read more about health and social care scandals and whistleblowing

Alder Hey Children's Hospital

A public inquiry in 1999 revealed that Alder Hey Children's Hospital in Liverpool, United Kingdom (UK), retained patients' organs without family consent, particularly the heart of children who had died following cardiac surgery. The official report, following investigation into this scandal, the *Redfern Report* was published in 2001 and resulted in public outcry and many suits filed with the High Court against NHS hospitals for removing the body parts of dead patients without consent. As a result, the *Human Tissue Act* came into force in 2004, which provides a legislative framework for issues relating to body and organ donation. The *Human Tissue Act (2004)* can be viewed at www.legislation.gov.uk/ukpga/2004/30/contents

Winterbourne View abuse

The Winterbourne View scandal, exposed by the BBC Panorama programme in 2011, revealed shocking undercover footage of repeated abuse of residents of a private residential home that specialised in care for people with learning disabilities. It led to a government pledge to move all people with learning disabilities and/or autism inappropriately placed in such institutions into community care. Despite several safeguarding concerns being raised by the staff , allegations were not investigated before the programme aired.

Following the programme, several arrests were made, and the Care Quality Commission (CQC) admitted that it recognised that '...there were indications of problems at this hospital, which should have led to us taking action sooner' (Care Quality Commission 2011). Winterbourne View was closed later in 2011, with every effort made to ensure minimal disruption to residents who needed to be moved to alternative services. Eleven staff admitted charges of neglect and ill treatment of residents, and six received custodial sentences. Two nurses involved were removed from the Nursing and Midwifery Council register.

A summary of the Government Response to this scandal can be found at https://assets.publishing.service.gov.uk/government/uploads/system/uploads/attachment_data/file/213221/4-page-summary.pdf

Maternity services

The *Ockenden Review*, a major report into maternity scandal at Shrewsbury and Telford NHS Trust, investigated failings in maternity care. The investigation initially began in 2017 when an independent was asked to investigate 23 cases of concern at Shrewsbury and Telford NHS Trust. The review involved the examination of more than 1,800 cases of harm, including unnecessary deaths of babies and mothers, and babies left with lasting brain damage. It found that there was a lack of kindness or compassion towards families affected from staff within the Trust. It is thought that a culture to keep caesarean section rates low may have been a contributory factor, and a whistleblower who worked at the Trust referred to 'a climate of fear' among staff members who were reluctant to report concerns because of the risk of bullying and victimisation.

The Trust took full responsibility for the failings in care and has offered an apology for the distress and hurt caused.

Following the inquiry into the UK's biggest maternity services scandal, the then Health Secretary, Sajid Javid, apologised to the families affected and pledged to hold those responsible to account. The report made a range of recommendations for the local trust, the wider NHS and for the government, aimed at improving the quality of maternity services across the UK.

A summary of findings, conclusions and essential actions recommended following this scandal can be found at www.gov.uk/government/publications/final-report-of-the-ockenden-review/ockenden-review-summary-of-findings-conclusions-and-essential-actions.

Activity 5.8: Do you know how to raise concerns within your organisation?

What action would you take if you witnessed abuse or sub-standard practice in your workplace? Would you know how to raise concerns if you did witness poor practice? Also, reflect on how you would have felt if you worked as a health and social care professional in any of the care organisations affected by high-profile scandals. Even if you were personally unaware of the situations, what questions might these scandals raise about professionalism, responsibility, accountability and raising concerns?

Candour

According to the Nursing and Midwifery Council (2018), duty of candour is about being open and honest—the values the public expect of any H&SC professional. There are two types of duty of candour: statutory and professional (Care Quality Commission 2021).

It is clear from previous accounts of poor care that, in the past, candour has not always been upheld. Before 2014, there was no legal obligation to share information when healthcare provision had been negligent, but the Francis Inquiry (Francis 2013) recommended the introduction of statutory duty of candour.

Applying duty of candour in practice has implications for public protection and patient-centred care because it is essential that the patient, as well as their family, carer or advocate, are kept informed about the patient's care, even if care delivery has been sub-optimal or a mistake has been made.

According to the Care Quality Commission (2021), an apology is a key part of duty of candour: 'you must apologise for the harm caused, regardless of fault, as well as being open and transparent about what has happened.' It is also essential that mistakes are highlighted as soon as possible and that individuals and teams are encouraged to discuss 'near miss' incidents that had the potential to result in harm to learn from them and are not discouraged from raising concerns (Nursing and Midwifery Council and General Medical Council 2022). The main way to ensure a duty of candour is upheld is by developing an organisational culture that promotes learning from mistakes and not blame and by creating an environment that promotes reflection and learning from mistakes to improve future practice and prevent harmful errors.

Interprofessional education or learning

Inter-professional education (IPE) or inter-professional learning (IPL) is a complex area of professional activity on which there is a large body of research and guidance. There is no adequate space here to explore it fully. Briefly, IPE is defined as: '...occur[ing] when two or more professions learn about, from and with each other to enable effective collaboration and improve health outcomes' (World Health Organization 2010).

The authors of a systematic review (Reeves *et al.* 2013) on the effectiveness of IPE interventions compared with no educational interventions in H&SC settings found that, of the 15 studies included, seven reported positive outcomes for IPE in areas such as diabetes care and patient satisfaction. Four studies reported mixed outcomes, and four studies reported no impact on professional practice or patient care. The authors maintain that:

> While uniprofessional education remains the dominant model for delivering education for health and social care professionals, IPE is increasingly becoming common. Advocacy and implementation of IPE reflects the premise that IPE will contribute to developing healthcare providers with the skills and knowledge needed to work in a collaborative manner (p.15).

On programmes with students working in diverse clinical settings, IPL can occur naturally to some degree in and out of the classroom. You should avail yourself of all IPL opportunities.

Self-evaluation and reflection: An ongoing process

Reflection is a paramount activity in H&SC education and practice. What is reflection? The Health and Care Professions Council (2023) defines it as:

> ...the thought process where individuals consider their experiences to gain insights about their whole practice. Reflection supports individuals to continually improve the way they work or the quality of care they give to people. It is a familiar, continuous and routine part of the work of health and care professionals.

The HCPC also notes that, while reflection takes many different forms, it is important to understand that activities linked to reflection are not themselves reflective. Reflecting is not simply about talking or writing about the working day, but these activities become reflective when drawn on to assess practice and develop professional learning (Health and Care Professions Council 2021).

Reflection is a professional requirement of NMC registration and revalidation and referred to in the codes and standards of other regulatory bodies. The NMC Code states that: 'We want to encourage nurses, midwives and nursing associates to reflect on their practice, so they can identify any improvements or changes to their practice as a result of what they have learnt' (Nursing and Midwifery Council 2021a). Reflection is, therefore, important at all stages of a H&SC professional's career: during initial training, once fully qualified and during preceptorship (see below) and when seeking revalidation.

Looking after yourself

Reflection can be facilitated by using a framework such as the widely used one developed by Graham Gibbs (Gibbs 1988). Gibbs' reflective framework asks those reflecting to think (honestly and deeply) about their emotional responses to real-world experiences and—alongside analysis of the experience more generally—to consider how'd they behave and what actions they'd take if they encountered the same or a similar event again.

Practitioner learner reflective accounts sometimes describe feelings of apprehension, uncertainty and even fear, especially when dealing with novel or challenging experiences under stressful working conditions. Student action plans arising from these reflections often refer to the need to look after oneself, to be mindful of the impact of such experiences on physical and emotional health.

The issue of self-care is an important one; understanding the need for self-care should begin from the earliest days of an H&SC professional's career, from initial training and education to retirement. What exactly is self-care? The World Health Organization (World Health Organization 2022) defines it as: '…the ability of individuals, families and communities to promote health, prevent disease, maintain health and cope with illness and disability with or without the support of a healthcare provider'. As this definition suggests, self-care is about coping with ill health (with or without professional input), and it's also about developing strategies to manage day-to-day stresses, an ever-present feature of most H&SC settings which are often short-staffed and under-resourced.

Self-care is a broad term that relates to diverse aspects of people's lives such as looking after basic hygiene needs, eating a balanced diet and getting enough exercise. It's also about recognising the signs that you may be becoming stressed or unwell and implementing coping strategies. Some obvious examples of becoming stressed include being less tolerant of others, being short-tempered, losing your appetite (or over-eating), not sleeping properly, feeling run-down and tired and misusing alcohol or other substances.

As well as identifying your own early warning signs of stress, it's important that you are aware of things that 'trigger' stress. Being aware of your own triggers may help you avoid them. However, this may not always be possible, hence the need to be aware of what helps you cope when you are feeling stressed. Importantly, what works for one person may not work for another. It's important to develop your own self-care strategies and to make others aware of these so that they can assist you in managing your well-being.

Panel 5.4: What causes you stress and what keeps you well?

Spend a few moments thinking about what causes you stress in your personal and professional life and what helps keeps you well.

You might, for example, think that some aspects of family life are stressful (caring for babies and young children is rewarding but can be challenging). It might be work that causes most stress; maybe you have a high workload, or you don't feel as well supported by colleagues as you should be.

What things help keep you well? Talking to loved ones? Sharing stories with colleagues? Playing sports or exercising? Taking holidays?

Panel 5.5: Self-care strategies

Common self-care strategies include:

- Being mindful: This involves: '…paying attention to what is going on inside and outside ourselves, moment by moment' (NHS 2022). Watch the video from Every Mind Matters (https://youtu.be/wfDTp2GogaQ) to learn more about this practice

- Taking care of physical health needs: are you getting enough sleep? Is your diet healthy? Are you getting enough exercise? Walking in natural, green spaces is especially beneficial for mental and physical health
- Challenging negative thinking: Our thoughts are like reflexes; they just pop into our heads, and we feel like we have little control over them. However, we can challenge our negative thought processes. See MindWell (2023) for tips on how to do this
- Being prepared: A lot of stress relates to feeling unprepared. Studying on an H&SC programme can be intense, more so than many other degree programmes, as it's completed alongside work in clinical settings. In addition, many H&SC students are mature and looking after family members. Practical things to do to be more prepared include being aware of submission dates; giving yourself time to make changes to essays and reports; not leaving submission to the last minute, as this is a cause of stress for most students; and setting small but achievable goals to ensure that work is completed on time. Remember to seek help from academic staff if you are struggling with assignments; most tutors will offer tutorials to learners in need of additional help
- Seeking help from a professional: There may be times when seeking professional help is necessary. Students can approach student services in their university or college for referral to counselling. Students who are also H&SC workers can access help in their workplace. More information about professional and other sources of help for H&SC workers can be seen at www.england.nhs.uk/support ing-our-nhs-people/support-now/.

Registration as a health and social care professional: New role and new responsibilities

Registration as a professional with the relevant regulatory body can be a time of great happiness and excitement but also trepidation. Adjusting to a new role can be emotional and physically tiring. Newly qualified professionals might be uncertain about the boundaries of their practice, concerned about the acquisition of new responsibilities and anxious to prove their worth in the workplace. H&SC workers are very dependent on the support of others during this time. How best can this be done?

Preceptorship

Preceptorship is what's called a 'structured start' for newly qualified practitioners (NHS England 2022b). The Nursing and Midwifery Council (2022b) observes that newly registered practitioners have the knowledge and other attributes to join the NMC register, and preceptorship then offers:

…the structured support needed for new nurses, midwives and nursing associates to successfully convert this knowledge into everyday practice…The preceptorship period provides the basis for the beginning of a lifelong journey of reflection, and the ability to self-identify continuing professional development needs… (p.5).

The NHS England (2022) has described five principles of preceptorship. These are focused around organisational culture, the quality and oversight of preceptorship, the empowerment of preceptees, preparation of preceptors for their role and the preceptorship programme itself (which can vary in length and content according to the needs of the new registrant).

What happens when things don't go to plan?

Most mistakes in H&SC settings are minor, do not have lasting impacts and can usually be resolved 'in-house' through informal or formal processes.

Very occasionally, however, an H&SC worker's ability to practise is questioned because of an error, their behaviour or a lapse in practice. What happens next depends on the professional concerned, the nature of the mistake, the strength of the evidence about the incident and whether or not the practitioner has learnt from the mistake.

In this section, we will look at the NMC's process of dealing with midwives, nurses and nursing associates whose ability to practise is called into question.

Fitness to Practise and NMC hearings

The NMC's Fitness to Practise process reflects its regulatory role, which involves:

> …investigating concerns about nurses, midwives and nursing associates—something that affects a tiny minority of professionals each year. Our standards are set out in The Code … If they [nurse, midwife or nursing associate] meet these standards, this is what we call being fit to practise. If someone raises a concern about someone's skills, behaviour and their right to be on our register, this will go through … the fitness to practise process. This process allows us to understand… whether a registered professional presents a risk to the public (Nursing and Midwifery Council 2022a).

Panel 5.6: Nursing and Midwifery Councils' 12 principles for fitness to practise

1. Fitness to practise is person-centred
2. Fitness to practise is about the management of future risk, not punishment for past events
3. Protection patients and the public is helped by making fitness to practise decisions swiftly and publishing the decisions openly
4. Employers should act first to deal with concerns about a registered practitioner unless the risk to others is so serious that immediate action is warranted
5. Regulatory action is necessary when there's a risk to patient safety that an employer isn't effectively managing
6. The context in which the practitioner was practising is taken into account when deciding whether there's a risk to patient safety
7. There may be no need to take regulatory action for a clinical mistake, even where there has been serious harm, if there's no longer a risk to patient safety and the practitioner can demonstrate learning from the experience

8. Deliberately covering up when things go wrong will result in restrictive regulatory action
9. In cases about clinical practice, action is likely to be needed only if the regulatory concern can't be addressed
10. In cases that aren't about clinical practice, action is likely to be needed only if the concerns raise fundamental questions about the trustworthiness of the professional
11. Some regulatory concerns can't be addressed and require restrictive regulatory action
12. Hearings resolve central aspects of a case that the Nursing and Midwifery Council and the practitioner don't agree on.

Adapted from: Nursing and Midwifery Council (2022b).

Activity 5.9: What kind of things can lead to the expression of a concern about a Nursing and Midwifery Council registrant?

Common errors or causes for concern that might lead to the expression of a concern include:

- Inadequate record keeping
- Medication errors
- Not adhering to professional boundaries
- Actions that result in patient harm
- Fraud
- Misconduct

Once a concern about an NMC registered professional has been raised, a process of 'screening' then takes place. This process has three stages:

1. Is there a written concern about a nurse, midwife or nursing associate on the NMC register?
2. Is there evidence of a concern that could warrant regulatory action to protect the public?
3. Is there evidence to show that the nurse, midwife or nursing associate is currently fit to practise?

Depending on the outcome of screening, the H&SC worker may be allowed to continue to practise or subjected to a restriction on their ability to work in an H&SC setting. In some cases, screening leads to a full investigation. This can result in a number of outcomes including meetings and hearings.

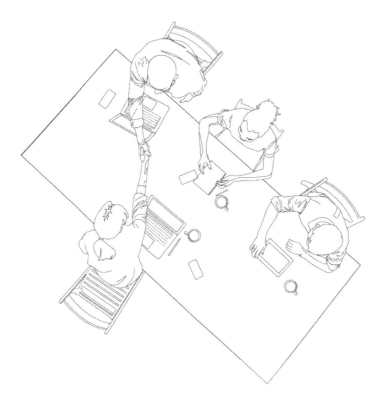

Figure 5.2 Nursing and Midwifery Council Hearing
Image credit: Tamsin Arai Drake

Panel 5.7: Read some Nursing and Midwifery Council hearing reports

Go to the NMC website and look at some recent NMC hearing reports to see the types of concerns that lead to hearings and what sanctions were applied: www.nmc.org.uk/concerns-nurses-midwives/hearings/hearings-sanctions/.

It is rare for a professional to be asked to attend a hearing, as these occur only in the most serious cases. Of more than 700,000 practitioners the NMC regulates, nearly 1,800 referrals from employers were received during 2019–2020. Of these, 62% progressed to the investigation stage, and only 7% progressed to a hearing (Nursing and Midwifery Council 2021b).

Summary

This chapter examined what it means to be an H&SC professional by discussing professional attributes and identities and examining concepts such as accountability, candour, safeguarding, person-centred care, reflection and self-care. All registered professionals begin a period of preceptorship in the initial post-registration period when newly quali-fied practitioners' activities and behaviours are regulated by governing bodies such as the NMC. We also discussed the NMC's Fitness to Practise process. This is a highly structured approach to investigating concerns about a registrant but is a rare occurrence. Most concerns are minor and are usually resolved through in-house processes.

Box 5.4: Key learning points

- Professionalism is associated with words and terms such as 'trust', 'expertise', 'reliability', 'respect' and 'accountability'
- Key concepts relevant to an examination of professionalism include person-centred care and safeguarding
- The public need to have confidence and trust in care professionals if effective, therapeutic relationships are to be developed
- Whistleblowers are workers who report wrong-doing in their workplaces, and they are protected in law
- Your behaviour at work is judged against professional codes of practice
- You have a duty of candour and a responsibility to raise concerns about any indi-viduals or organisations delivering sub-standard care or services
- Registration as a professional can be a time of great happiness, but adjusting to a new role can present challenges
- Most mistakes in care settings are minor and can usually be resolved 'in-house' through informal or formal processes.

References

BALTHAZARD, C., 2015. *What does it mean to be a professional?* [viewed 23 June 2022]. *HRPA series on professionalization, professionalism, and ethics for human resources.* Available from: https://hrpa.s3.amazonaws.com/uploads/2020/10/What-it-means-to-be-a-professional.pdf

BENNETT, C. L., A. H. JAMES and D. KELLY, 2020. Beyond tropes: Towards a new image of nursing in the wake of COVID-19. *Journal of clinical nursing*, 29(15-16), 2753-2755. https://doi.org/10.1111/jocn.15346

BROTHERTON, G. and S. PARKER, 2013. *Your foundation in health and social care.* London: Sage Publications Ltd.

CARE QUALITY COMMISSION, 2011. *CQC statement on Panorama's investigation* [viewed 23 December 2022]. Available from: www.cqc.org.uk/news/releases/cqc-statement-panorama%E2%80%99s-investigation

CARE QUALITY COMMISSION, 2021. *Regulation 20: Duty of candour* [viewed 23 December 2022]. Available from: www.cqc.org.uk/guidance-providers/regulations-enforcement/regulation-20-duty-candour

CAULFIELD, H., 2005. *Vital notes for nurses: accountability.* Malden: Blackwell Publishing.

CAZA, B. and S. J. CREARY, 2016. The construction of professional identity. In: A. WILKINSON, D., HISLOP and C. COUPLAND, eds. *Perspectives on contemporary professional work: Challenges and experiences.* Cheltenham, UK: Edward Elgar Publishing, pp.259-285.

CUMMINGS, J. and V. BENNETT, 2012. *Compassion in practice: Nursing midwifery and care staff: Our vision and strategy.* NHS Commissioning Board: Crown copyright.

FRANCIS, R., 2013. *Report of the Mid Staffordshire NHS Foundation Trust Public Inquiry.* London: The Stationary Office.

GALLAGHER, A. and S. HODGE, 2012. *Ethics, law and Professional issues: A practice–based approach for health professionals.* Basingstoke: Palgrave McMillan.

GIBBS, G., 1988. *Learning by doing: A guide to teaching and learning methods.* Further Education Unit. Oxford Polytechnic: Oxford.

HEALTH AND CARE PROFESSIONS COUNCIL, 2021. *Benefits of becoming a reflective practitioner* [viewed 06 May 2023]. Available from: www.hcpc-uk.org/standards/meeting-our-standards/reflective-practice/what-is-reflection/

HEALTH AND CARE PROFESSIONS COUNCIL, 2021. *Confidentiality and accountability* [viewed 25 September 2022]. Available from: www.hcpc-uk.org/standards/meeting-our-standards/confidentiality/guidance-on-confidentiality/confidentiality-and-accountability/

HEALTH EDUCATION ENGLAND, 2017. *The nursing associate curriculum framework.* Leeds: Health Education England.

KITWOOD, T., 1997. *Dementia reconsidered: The person comes first.* Buckingham: Open University Press.

MINDWELL, 2023. *Challenging negative thinking* [viewed 20 January 2023]. Available from: www.mindwell-leeds.org.uk/myself/exploring-your-mental-health/depression/challenging-negative-thinking/

NEARY, S., 2014. *Professional identity: What I call myself defines who I am* (Career Matters, Issue 2.3) [viewed 25 September 2022]. Available from: https://core.ac.uk/download/pdf/46170813.pdf

NHS, 2022. *Mindfulness* [viewed 20 January 2023]. Available from: www.nhs.uk/mental-health/self-help/tips-and-support/mindfulness/

NHS ENGLAND, 2019. *Safeguarding children, young people and adults at risk in the NHS: Safeguarding accountability and assurance framework* [viewed 25 September 2022]. Available from: www.england.nhs.uk/wp-content/uploads/2015/07/safeguarding-children-young-people-adults-at-risk-saaf-1.pdf)

NHS ENGLAND, 2022a. *Freedom to speak up–annual report on whistleblowing disclosures made to us by NHS workers* [viewed 25 September 2022]. Available from: www.england.nhs.uk/ourwork/freedom-to-speak-up/whistleblowing-disclosures/

NHS ENGLAND, 2022b. *National preceptorship framework for nursing* [viewed 25 September 2022]. Available from: www.england.nhs.uk/long-read/national-preceptorship-framework-for-nursing/

NURSING AND MIDWIFERY COUNCIL, 2018. *The code: Professional standards of practice and behaviour for nurses, midwives and nursing associates* [viewed 25 September 2022]. Available from: www.nmc.org.uk/standards/code/

NURSING AND MIDWIFERY COUNCIL, 2021a. *Written reflective accounts* [viewed 25 September 2022]. Available from: www.nmc.org.uk/revalidation/requirements/written-reflective-accounts/

NURSING AND MIDWIFERY COUNCIL, 2021b. *Managing concerns: A resource for employers* [viewed 25 September 2022]. Available from: www.nmc.org.uk/employer-resource/introduction-managing-concerns/overview/

NURSING AND MIDWIFERY COUNCIL, 2022a. *An introduction to fitness to practise: A step-by-step guide to our fitness to practise* [viewed 25 September 2022]. Available from: www.nmc.org.uk/concerns-nurses-midwives/what-is-fitness-to-practise/an-introduction-to-fitness-to-practise/

NURSING AND MIDWIFERY COUNCIL, 2022b. *Our fitness to practise aims and objectives* [viewed 25 September 2022]. Available from: www.nmc.org.uk/concerns-nurses-midwives/what-is-fitness-to-practise/an-introduction-to-fitness-to-practise/our-fitness-to-practise-aims-and-objectives/

NURSING AND MIDWIFERY COUNCIL and GENERAL MEDICAL COUNCIL, 2022. *Openness and honesty when things go wrong: The professional duty of candour* (joint guidance with the General Medical Council on the duty of candour) [viewed 25 September 2022]. Available from: www.nmc.org.uk/globalassets/sitedocuments/nmc-publications/openness-and-honesty-professional-duty-of-candour.pdf

PEATE, I., 2019. *Learning to care: The nursing associate.* London: Elsevier Ltd.

REEVES, S. *et al.*, 2013. Interprofessional education: Effects on professional practice and healthcare outcomes. *Cochrane database of systematic reviews*, 2013(3), CD002213. https://doi.org/10.1002/14651858.CD002213.pub3

ROSS, H., A. M. TOD and A. CLARKE, 2014. Understanding and achieving person-centred care: The nurse perspective. *Journal of clinical nursing*, 24(9-10), 1223-1233. https://doi.org/10.1111/jocn.12662

ROYAL COLLEGE OF NURSING, 2022. *Accountability and delegation* [viewed 25 September 2022]. Available from: www.rcn.org.uk/Professional-Development/Accountability-and-delegation/Accountability-and-delegation-case-studies

SAVAGE, J. and L. MOORE, 2004. *Interpreting accountability: An ethnographic study of practice nurses, accountability and multidisciplinary team decision-making in the context of clinical governance.* Oxford: RCN Institute.

TEN HOEVE, Y., G. JANSEN and P. ROODBOL, 2014. The nursing profession: Public image, self-concept and professional identity. A discussion paper. *Journal of advanced nursing*, 70(2), 295-309. https://doi.org/10.1111/jan.12177

WORLD HEALTH ORGANIZATION, 2010. *Framework for action on interprofessional education and collaborative practice* [viewed 25 September 2022]. Available from: http://apps.who.int/iris/bitstream/handle/10665/70185/WHO_HRH_HPN_10.3_eng.pdf?sequence=1&isAllowed=y

WORLD HEALTH ORGANIZATION, 2022. *Self-care interventions for health* [viewed 20 January 2023]. Available from: www.who.int/news-room/fact-sheets/detail/self-care-health-interventions

6 Working with others
Supervision and mentoring

Gemma Burley and Lisa Arai

Box 6.1: Contents

- Introduction
- The professional and organisational context
- Teaching and learning theories: An overview
- Educational roles within health and social care
- Drawing on your own experiences of supervision and mentoring

---

Box 6.2: Learning outcomes

By the end of this chapter, you should be able to

- Define what supervision and mentoring are
- Discuss the different theories about how people learn
- Understand the diversity of mentoring roles within health and social care
- Reflect on the use of your own experience in your studies.

Box 6.3: Keywords

- Supervision
- Mentoring
- Nursing and Midwifery Council
- NHS Constitution for England
- Humanistic Learning Theory
- Andragogy
- Standards for Student Supervision and Assessment
- Coach
- CLIP (Collaborative Learning in Practice)
- GROW (Goals, Reality, Options and Will)

DOI: 10.4324/9781003198338-8

Introduction

Supervision, mentoring and teamwork play a vital role in health and social care (H&SC) practitioners' day-to-day, working life. There is no one definition of supervision or mentoring within healthcare, and definitions can differ between clinical areas or professions. One definition of supervision is that by the Health and Care Professions Council (HCPC) (Health and Care Professions Council 2022), where the Council says supervision is: '...a process or professional learning and development that enables individuals to reflect on and develop their knowledge, skills, and competence, through agreed and regular support with another professional'. Burgess, Diggele and Mellis (2018) describe mentorship as '... a process though which an experienced person (mentor) guides another (mentee) in developing skills and knowledge for their professional development' (p.197).

In the United Kingdom (UK), as part of their continuing professional development and to meet future workforce planning needs, H&SC workers are required to assume the role of both a student and a teacher throughout their career. With an institution as complex as the National Health Service (NHS), which involves working within specialist teams and in wider multi-disciplinary teams, a sound knowledge of supervision and mentoring, and the challenges associated with this, is necessary for all H&SC professionals.

This chapter discusses supervision and mentoring within professional H&SC settings, considers theories of how people learn, explores educational roles within H&SC and examines how you can draw on your own experiences of supervision and mentoring in your studies. This is a vast subject on which there is a large body of research and guidance, and this chapter is an introduction only. You are strongly advised to read around this topic.

The professional and organisational context

Healthcare careers are usually governed by professional bodies associated with the individual's profession (see chapter 4). The Nursing and Midwifery Council (NMC) and HCPC both set out codes describing the importance of supervision, assessment and mentoring of others in the workplace (Nursing and Midwifery Council 2018a; Health and Care Professions Council 2017).

Standards for student supervision and assessment

In both its code and its Standards for Student Supervision and Assessment (SSSA), the NMC outlines the role that registered nurses, midwives and nursing associates should take in the supervision of others, advising that it is the responsibility of these professionals to act as role models and share knowledge and expertise with others (Nursing and Midwifery Council 2018b).

The SSSA, introduced in September 2018, fundamentally changed the way student nurses, midwives and nursing associates are supported in practice and the role that registered professionals play in students' learning (Nursing and Midwifery Council 2018a). The SSSA moved away from previous roles such as 'mentor' and 'mentee' and introduced the roles of practice assessor (PA), practice supervisor (PS) and academic assessor (AA) (see Nursing and Midwifery Council 2018a for detailed information on these three roles). This move from individual mentorship to the tripartite support of

PA/PS/AA reflects the idea that student support and supervision is every H&SC registrant's responsibility.

Health and Care Professions Council

The HCPC's Standards of Education and Training (Health and Care Professions Council 2017) set out the requirements of registered HCPC professionals who are supporting students in practice. This covers support of those on educational programmes and support of students/colleagues in practice. Students undertaking practice-based learning must do so in a safe and effective learning environment and be offered adequate support by colleagues. This support includes that provided by practice educators who are defined by the HCPC as 'a person who is responsible for a learner's education during their practice-based learning' (Health and Care Professions Council 2020).

Organisational contexts

While H&SC professionals usually work within the codes, or according to the standards, of their individual governing bodies (NMC/HCPC/General Medical Council etc.), they also work within organisational contexts. These could be individual Trusts, general practice surgeries or residential care homes. H&SC workers also work within the broader NHS organisational context and must adhere to its principles and values. The NHS Constitution for England describes these as they apply to England and sets out the rights to which patients and others are entitled (Department of Health and Social Care 2021). There are seven guiding principles in this constitution (see Panel 6.1).

Panel 6.1: National Health Service (NHS) guiding principles

- The NHS provides a comprehensive service, available to all
- Access to NHS services is based on clinical need not ability to pay
- The NHS aspires to the highest standards of excellence and professionalism
- The patient will be at the heart of everything the NHS does
- The NHS works across organisational boundaries
- The NHS is committed to providing the best value for taxpayers' money
- The NHS is accountable to the public, communities and patients it serves.

Effective supervision, mentoring and teamwork underpin these guiding principles (especially: 'The NHS aspires to the highest standards of excellence and professionalism' and 'The patient will be at the heart of everything the NHS does'). To ensure that patients receive the highest standards of care, H&SC professionals need to engage in career-long learning, and supervision and mentoring is central to this.

We've been concerned thus far primarily with broader organisational contexts. As noted briefly above, there are Trust or other organisation-specific values and principles that H&SC professionals must work within. Inevitably, these values differ across organisations, although all reflect the core NHS Constitution for England principles.

Activity 6.1: Find the Trust values of your local National Health Service Trust

Identify the Trust values of your local National Health Service Trust. What are they? Consider how they relate to the National Health Service constitution and their link to supervision, mentoring and teamwork.

Teaching and learning theories: an overview

Understanding how people acquire knowledge and learn is a key activity in any discussion of supervision and mentoring of others. Do all learners learn the same way? The short answer is 'No'. Recognising this and adapting supervision and mentoring to suit the needs of learners is imperative if students are to succeed. Aspects of learning to consider include people's individual learning style, their personal preferences and their previous experience.

Educational learning theory includes many perspectives including those associated with behaviourism, cognitivism, humanism and constructivism learning theory. While not an all-encompassing list, we will focus here on the salient elements of some of these theories and consider their application to H&SC professional education.

Humanistic Learning Theory/humanism

The Humanistic Learning Theory is a popular educational theory based on the idea of the learner being central to their own learning objectives and needs and where learners play an active role in their own education. Key theorists associated with the Humanistic Learning Theory include Abraham Maslow, who created the famous hierarchy of needs (Maslow 1943) and Carl Rogers. Their research became the foundation of the Humanistic Learning Theory. This maintains that everyone has a natural potential for learning and teachers should be facilitators of this potential but should be guided by the learners while doing so.

Andragogy

Andragogy is a key theory within humanism and relates to the study of how adults learn. Pedagogy is derived from the ancient Greek 'leading children', while andragogy refers to 'leading man' and can be referred to as 'the art and science of teaching adults'. A key theorist in the field of andragogy, Malcolm Knowles (Knowles 1984), described five assumptions for adult learning (see Panel 6.2).

Panel 6.2: Knowles' five assumptions for adult learning

1. As a person matures, they become more independent and self-directed in their learning; they want to have ownership over it
2. Adults bring experience to the learning process. It's important for teachers to understand the scope and extent of this experience

3. Children absorb everything as they grow, but adult learners are more selective about the information they receive
4. Adult learners don't necessarily want to learn everything about a concept; they want to understand how to apply that concept to problem solving
5. Adult learners are motivated by internal factors rather than external ones

Adapted from: Knowles (1984).

These assumptions were based on the principle that adult learners need to be in control of their own learning.

Over the years, there has been some dispute among educational theorists about the relevance and application of Knowles' five assumptions. This includes by Knowles himself, who began to change his view of andragogy versus pedagogy and, instead, likened learning to a spectrum between teacher-driven and learner-driven but taking into account the importance of seeing students as an individual with individual learning needs and desires (Merriam, Cafferella and Baumgartner 2007).

Behaviourism

The Behaviourist Learning Theory centres on the idea that all behaviours are learnt through people's interactions with the environment throughout their life. Behaviourism maintains that learning occurs in response to specific stimuli, resulting in conditioning. Initially developed by psychologist John B. Watson, Ivan Pavlov and B. F. Skinner popularised this theory by focusing on the concept of conditioning and describing two forms of conditioning: classical and operant (Staddon 2021).

Classical conditioning

Detailed research on classical conditioning was first conducted by Ivan Pavlov, whose famous experiments with dogs examined how stimuli causes an involuntary response. His experiments showed that dogs could be taught to salivate at the sound of a bell if the bell was associated with food. Pavlov noted that the dogs would initially salivate at the sight of food but would not respond to the sound of a bell. However, after repeatedly ringing a bell at the same time as presenting food, Pavlov was able to teach dogs to salivate at the sound of the bell even in the absence of food. This experiment showed that new behaviours could be taught (i.e., the subject could be 'conditioned' to learn new behaviours).

Operant conditioning

The concept of classical conditioning was further developed by B. F. Skinner (Staddon 2021). Skinner accepted the idea of classical conditioning. However, he believed it to be too simplistic when seeking to understand human behaviour and learning. Skinner's development of the concept of operant conditioning focused on the idea of behaviour being conditioned via positive and negative stimuli to promote a voluntary response. This is different from the involuntary response seen with classical conditioning.

One of his most famous experiments in the field of operant conditioning included the conditioning of animals (specifically rats and pigeons) in his 'Skinner boxes'. Animals placed in these boxes were conditioned to produce a certain behaviour in response to either positive or negative stimuli. For example, a rat placed in the box could learn that, by pressing a lever, it could receive food (positive reinforcement) or stop a loud sound (negative reinforcement). Skinner concluded that positive reinforcement had a longer lasting effect than negative reinforcement (that is, the behaviour is more likely to be repeated from a positive response than from a negative response). He also concluded that negative reinforcement could produce a counter-productive response.

Cognitivism

Cognitivism focuses on how information is received, processed and organised within the mind. Its core belief is that learning centres around gathering of all relevant information to build a complete picture and behavioural modification comes from this thought processing. One of the key theorists of cognitivism was Jean Piaget (Piaget 1929) who developed the theory of the four stages of cognitive development. This theory examined the development of children's cognitive abilities and proposed that, as a child grows, their cognitive abilities develop and change.

As a theoretical framework, cognitivism was borne out of dissatisfaction with behaviourist explanations for human learning and behaviour. While behaviourism acknowledged the notion of cognition, this was considered a behaviour. Cognitivists argued that cognition played a key role in behaviour and thought processes, and this differed from person-to-person. Therefore, from a cognitivist perspective, cognition could not be simply labelled a behaviour which could be conditioned.

Bloom's taxonomy

Bloom's taxonomy (Bloom *et al.* 1956) is a model classifying the cognitive processes of students at different levels (see also chapter 2). The model refers to cognitive, affective and psychomotor domains. The cognitive domain focuses on the thinking skills of students, classifying their skills depending on their ability to understand the subject matter. This ranges from the basic skill of remembering specific facts or details about a subject to more advanced skills, those involving the evaluation of a subject and those advancing a learner's ability to form an opinion on a specific issue. This model not only helps educators identify the cognitive level of their students but also provides a framework for students to develop their cognitive abilities to higher levels of understanding and analysis.

Educational roles within Health and Social Care

The development of the SSSA by the NMC introduced new roles within nursing and healthcare education (Nursing and Midwifery Council 2018b). The role of PA and PS encompassed several roles such as mentor, coach and role model used within practice to support student nurses, midwives and nursing assistants. While the terms PA/PS are new to healthcare education, their embodied roles have long been used by healthcare students and their teachers. The roles of a mentor and a coach will be discussed here.

Mentor

The term 'mentor' was the key person of support and learning used by the NMC in its support of students within practice (Nursing and Midwifery Council 2008). While this term has been replaced within nursing practice education, the role of a mentor still has a place within nursing education and in wider healthcare professionals' education. Mentors are seen as more experienced staff members who guide a mentee (with less experience) in developing specific knowledge and skills within the mentee's professional development. Mentors encompass several characteristics and roles to guide the mentees' development, such as teacher, guide and role model (Burgess, Diggele and Mellis 2018).

There has been much research and discussion about what makes an effective mentor for healthcare students (Bailey-McHale and Hart 2013), and while there is no definitive definition of the characteristics of an effective mentor, most have similar qualities (see Panel 6.3).

Panel 6.3: Characteristics of an effective mentor

An effective mentor should be:

- Patient
- Open-minded
- A role model
- Tactful
- Confident
- Approachable

Adapted from: Gopee (2015).

Research has also considered the effect of problematic or ineffective mentors on healthcare students. Darling (1986) called these mentors 'toxic' and split them into four categories (see Panel 6.4).

Panel 6.4: 'Toxic mentors'

1. Avoiders	Mentors who are not approachable, accessible or available
2. Dumpers	Dumpers deliberately expose students to experiences or situations the student is not prepared for, expecting a 'sink or swim' response
3. Blockers	These refuse to meet students' needs by refusing learning opportunities, withholding information or over-supervising the student
4. Destroyers/ criticisers	This kind of mentor destroys the student by belittling or undermining them in public or destroying their confidence

Adapted from: Darling (1986).

The effect of a poor mentor-mentee relationship can have a detrimental effect on student experience within healthcare and can lead to students leaving healthcare programmes (Jack *et al.* 2018).

It is possible for students in healthcare placements to encounter mentors with the above traits; however, it is not easy to explain why these mentors exist. The reasons for ineffective mentoring are found at both a personal and an institutional level. Fear and knowledge can play an important part in the making of an effective or ineffective mentor. As mentors are held accountable and responsible for the actions of their students, they can struggle in allowing students to undertake tasks through fear of the consequences should something go wrong. A lack of knowledge of student's capabilities or expectations can also have a negative impact, with mentors expecting too much or too little from their students.

While both fear and knowledge can be considered important issues with mentorship, these personal emotions could be linked to wider, institutional-level issues. Staff shortages within the NHS are an ongoing issue. In 2022, there were approximately 100,000 vacancies across the NHS; 40,000 of these were nurse vacancies. This equates to approximately one in ten unfilled posts (The King's Fund 2022). This problem has been compounded by the ongoing COVID-19 pandemic, with staff members reporting feelings of work-related stress and burnout because of the pandemic (Gemine *et al.* 2021). These factors, and others, equate to what can be seen a difficult work environment, with current staff members struggling with the responsibilities they face and not having the time or resources to adequately support students. Research has indicated that nursing students can often feel devalued and demotivated by clinical placements; some students report that they are used primarily to fill rota gaps (Jack *et al.* 2018).

Activity 6.2: Case study: Anita

Let's now look at a case study about Anita. She's a third-year nursing student who is on placement. Read her story below. While reading it, consider why or how this situation arose and think about how you would resolve it.

Anita's story

Anita is a third-year nursing student. She is currently 2 weeks into her 8-week placement in a high-dependency unit in a large teaching hospital. Her goals for this placement revolve around increasing her leadership and independent working skills in preparation for her course completion in a 6-month time period. This week, Anita has been allocated to work with Martin as one of her practice supervisors.

Her first week during placement was uneventful. She had a good induction to the high-dependency unit and met other members of the team. She had not met Martin, as he had been on annual leave during her first week. During their first shift together, Martin advised Anita to shadow him during the shift. He completed all medication administration, paperwork and communications with other staff members. Anita felt slightly frustrated and bored, as she did not feel she could practise her skills and, instead, was just following Martin around. She did not say this to Martin, as she felt things would improve as the week progressed.

The following two shifts followed the same pattern, with Anita not undertaking any tasks and instead shadowing and observing Martin completing the tasks. Martin did not offer to explain the reasons behind his actions and, for the most part, acted like Anita was not present. At the end of the third day, Anita approached her practice assessor and reported that she felt completely useless and had not learnt anything from Martin in the last three shifts. Why has this situation arisen? How can it be resolved?

Martin is showing the characteristics of the 'Avoiders and dumpers' mentor type (Darling 1986). Why Martin shows these characteristics is unclear; however, it could be linked to personal or institutional issues as discussed above: Fear of letting go of tasks (personal) or lack of staff meaning limited time to support Anita (institutional).

The reasons why Martin acts as he does are important, but Anita's actions should also be scrutinised. At no point has she appeared to discuss her frustrations with Martin. Instead, she approached a colleague to discuss her problems. While there could be sound reasons for this, if there is an issue with a mentor, an important first step in addressing this is to first approach the mentor and raise concerns with him or her. Martin may not be aware of the impact of his actions on Anita. In fact, this situation may have been easily resolved if Anita had spoken to Martin first.

The role of a coach

Coaches have been widely used in different areas—in and outside healthcare—for several decades. Sports coaching is a well-known activity, with both team coaches and individual coaches used with most professional and amateur athletes to help athletes achieve their full potential. Roles such as a life coach and a business coach are also well known. However, the role of a coach has increasingly been used within healthcare education, with promising results. A coach's aim is to assist a learner in achieving specific goals by providing guidance and support to that learner. The Chartered Institute of Personnel and Development (Chartered Institute of Personnel and Development 2021) has usefully summarised some of the characteristics of a coach:

- The emphasis is on the learner developing their own solutions and actions
- The focus is on improving the performance and development of the learner
- Learners should have opportunities to better understand their own strengths and areas of improvement
- Activities have both individual and wider organisational goals
- The emphasis is on work performance
- Coaching is a skilled activity, which coaches should be trained to deliver

From this perspective, the emphasis in coaching is on students being responsible for their own learning. Learning should empower them; it is also seen as a key tool in preparing students to be independent practitioners upon graduation and after registration in their chosen profession. Within healthcare, coaching models such as Collaborative Learning in Practice (CLIP) and the GROW model have been used successfully in practice.

The Collaborative Learning in Practice model

The CLIP model of supporting learners in practice was first developed in the Netherlands and has been piloted across several NHS Trusts in the UK. The CLIP model has its basis as a coaching framework used in clinical practice, where students are encouraged to take a lead in their own learning through identified goals or learning outcomes. A set of students using CLIP would be expected to lead care for a specific set of patients during a shift. Peer support is paramount with the CLIP model, with students expected to support each other in the placement. This is done with the support of a coach within the placement areas.

Hill, Woodward and Arthur (2020) evaluated the CLIP model and acknowledged that some of the issues students may face in clinical practice impact the learning environment, such as staffing issues, patient complexities, busy clinical areas and staff skill mix. However, the CLIP model was considered advantageous for students in a number of ways if successfully implemented. It helped students develop leadership skills and confidence and boosted knowledge.

The GROW model

The GROW coaching model is often advocated as a coaching framework (Gopee 2015). The GROW model stands for 'Goals, Reality, Option and Will' and is a simple four-step framework for goal setting developed by Whitmore (1992). The GROW model is advocated for its simplicity and goal-related focus and can be used throughout a healthcare student's journey.

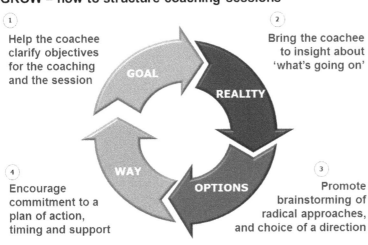

GROW – how to structure coaching sessions

1. Help the coachee clarify objectives for the coaching and the session

GOAL

2. Bring the coachee to insight about 'what's going on'

REALITY

4. Encourage commitment to a plan of action, timing and support

WAY

OPTIONS

3. Promote brainstorming of radical approaches, and choice of a direction

Adapted with permission from *The Tao of Coaching*, Max Landsberg, 1996

Figure 6.1 The GROW coaching model

Activity 6.3: Using the GROW model

The GROW model can be used for both personal and professional goals. Certain questions should be asked at each stage. These can help you identify realistic and achievable goals.

- Goal: what would you like to achieve? Is there a time frame? What are the benefits?
- Reality: what is the current situation? Are there any possible obstacles/barriers to your goal?
- Options: what options do you have to help you achieve your goal? Are there any positives/negatives to these actions?
- Will/Way: when will you start? What will you do? How will you know you have achieved your goal?

Adapted from: Whitmore (1992).

Using the GROW model and the questions above, consider a goal you would like to achieve. This could be personal, professional or academic. For example, run a 5-kilometre race, achieve a certain grade in an exam or achieve a proficiency in practice.

Drawing on your own experiences of supervision and mentoring

Many H&SC programmes—especially those that are practice-based—include modules on supervision and mentoring. These are often assessed through submission of a reflective essay where the learner is asked to demonstrate understanding of the theories around supervision and mentoring and reflect on their own experience of being a supervisor or mentor. What kind of advice can be offered to students writing their assignments on this subject? Briefly below are three tips to consider when writing about own experiences of supervision and mentoring in assignments.

Three tips for writing assignments on supervision and mentoring

Linking theory to practice

Make sure that you clearly link theory to practice in your assignment. This is something that is relatively easily achieved in terms of supervision and mentoring because there are so many theories and concepts to draw on (this chapter has highlighted some of these). By making a *clear* link between theory and your own experience, you demonstrate understanding of the theory and its application in practice. For example, you could refer to andragogy (discussed above) when reflecting on how ready you were when learning a new skill.

Be aware of emotions

This subject can provoke strong emotions, and this can be something that you wish to discuss in your reflection. However, remember that even with reflection, your writing should remain as professional and objective as possible. It's fine to acknowledge that you were upset by something a mentor said or did, for example, but write about this in a detached, professional way and analyse why you were upset by it (after all, the mentor almost certainly did not intend to upset you—they may have done so unwittingly and failed to realise the effect their words or actions would have had) and what you've learnt from the experience. Rather than write: 'I cried and cried after Sam criticised my record keeping', write: 'Sam's feedback on my record-keeping were emotionally upsetting but, ultimately, this was a learning experience and led to changes in my practice'.

Consider your future practice

As a student, you may have had minimal experience of supporting others in practice. However, once qualified, it is likely that you will have a professional responsibility to support and supervise others in practice. This is likely to be a key feature of your career in H&SC. An important element of reflective practice is considering your own future practice. Given this, it's useful to reflect on your time as a mentee and consider how it will influence your role as a supervisor in the future. What worked well for you? What would you change?

Summary

This chapter explored diverse aspects of supervision and mentoring. Most H&SC professionals will be supervisors and mentors at different stages in their careers. This can present challenges but is an essential part of the job. The NMC and other organisations have developed frameworks (such as the SSSA) to help practitioners in these activities. There are many theories describing how people learn, such as behaviourism and andragogy, and a body of work on the attributes of an effective mentor. Models, such as CLIP and GROW, are useful in helping those coaching others. We also briefly examined how you can draw on your own experiences of supervision and mentoring in your academic work.

Box 6.4: Key learning points

- Most health and social care professionals will be supervisors and mentors at different stages in their careers
- The Nursing and Midwifery Council and other organisations have developed frameworks to help practitioners when supervising or mentoring others
- Theories, such as behaviourism, cognitivism and andragogy, explain how people learn
- The attributes of an effective mentor have been described. Effective mentors are role models and are approachable. These are different to 'toxic' mentors such as 'avoiders'—mentors who are not approachable, accessible or available to mentees

- CLIP and GROW are examples of successful coaching models
- Three tips for students writing reflective essays on this subject are link theory to practice, be mindful when writing about your emotions and consider your future practice.

References

BAILEY-MCHALE, J. and D. M. HART, 2013. *Mastering mentorship*. London: SAGE Publications.

BLOOM, B. S. *et al.*, 1956. *Taxonomy of educational objectives: The classification of educational goals*. New York: Longmans.

BURGESS, A., C. DIGGELE and C. MELLIS, 2018. Mentorship in the health professions: A review. *The clinical teacher*, 15(3), 197-202. https://doi.org/10.1111/tct.12756

CHARTERED INSTITUTE OF PERSONNEL AND DEVELOPMENT, 2021. *Coaching and mentoring* [viewed 23 August 2022]. Available from: www.cipd.co.uk/knowledge/fundamentals/people/development/coaching-mentoring-factsheet#6995

DARLING, L. A., 1986. What to do about toxic mentors. *Nurse educator*, 11(2), 29-30. https://doi.org/10.1097/00006223-198603000-00013

DEPARTMENT OF HEALTH AND SOCIAL CARE, 2021. *The NHS Constitution for England* [viewed 23 August 2022]. Available from: www.gov.uk/government/publications/the-nhs-constitution-for-england/the-nhs-constitution-for-england

GEMINE, R. *et al.*, 2021. Factors associated with work-related burnout in NHS staff during COVID-19: A cross-sectional mixed methods study. *BMJ open*, 2811(1), e042591. https://doi.org/10.1136/bmjopen-2020-042591

GOPEE, N., 2015. *Mentoring and supervision in healthcare*. 3rd ed. London: Sage Publications.

HEALTH AND CARE PROFESSIONS COUNCIL, 2017. *Standards of education and training* [viewed 23 August 2022]. Available from: www.hcpc-uk.org/standards/standards-relevant-to-education-and-training/set/

HEALTH AND CARE PROFESSIONS COUNCIL, 2020. *HCPC statement on student supervision* [viewed 23 August 2022]. Available from: www.hcpc-uk.org/about-us/corporate-governance/policies/statements/hcpc-statement-on-student-supervision/

HEALTH AND CARE PROFESSIONS COUNCIL, 2022. *What is supervision?* [viewed 23 August 2022]. Available from: www.hcpc-uk.org/standards/meeting-our-standards/supervision-leadership-and-culture/supervision/what-is-supervision/

HILL, R., M. WOODWARD and A. ARTHUR, 2020. Collaborative Learning in Practice (CLIP): Evaluation of a new approach to clinical learning. *Nurse education today*, 85, 104295. https://doi.org/10.1016/j.nedt.2019.104295

JACK, K. *et al.*, 2018. 'My mentor didn't speak to me for the first four weeks': Perceived unfairness experienced by nursing students in clinical practice settings. *Journal of clinical nursing*, 27(5–6), 929-938. https://doi.org/10.1111/jocn.14015

KNOWLES, M., 1984. *Andragogy in action. Applying modern principles of adult education*. San Francisco, CA: Jossey Bass.

LANDSBERG, M. 1996. *The Tao of coaching*. London: Profile Books

MASLOW, A. H., 1943. A theory of human motivation. *Psychological review*, 50, 370-396.

MERRIAM, S. B., R. S. CAFFARELLA and L. BAUMGARTNER, 2007. *Learning in adulthood*. 3rd ed. San Francisco, CA: Jossey-Bass.

NURSING AND MIDWIFERY COUNCIL, 2008. *Standards to support learning and assessment in practice* [viewed 13 February 2022]. Available from: www.nmc.org.uk/globalassets/sitedocuments/standards/nmc-standards-to-support-learning-assessment.pdf

NURSING AND MIDWIFERY COUNCIL, 2018a. *The code: Professional standards of practice and behaviour for nurses, midwives and nursing associates* [viewed 13 February 2022]. Available from: www.nmc.org.uk/standards/code/

NURSING AND MIDWIFERY COUNCIL, 2018b. *Standards for student supervision and assessment* [viewed 13 February 2022]. Available from www.nmc.org.uk/standards-for-education-and-training/standards-for-student-supervision-and-assessment/

PIAGET, J., 1929. *The child's conception of the world*. London: Routledge.

STADDON, J., 2021. *The new behaviorism*. 3rd ed. Milton Park: Taylor and Francis.

KING'S FUND, 2022. *Key facts and figures about the NHS* [viewed 13 February 2022]. Available from: www.kingsfund.org.uk/audio-video/key-facts-figures-nhs

WHITMORE, J., 1992. *Coaching for performance: The principles and practices of coaching and leadership* (People skills for professionals series). Boston: Nicholas Brealey.

Part 3

Patients and Service Users: At the Heart of Health and Social Care

7 The nuts and bolts of the human body

Gemma Burley and Mandy Lyons

Box 7.1: Contents

- Introduction
- Organisation of the body
- Different human systems and homeostasis
- Nervous system
- Cardiovascular system
- Blood vessels and the circulatory system
- Respiratory system
- Endocrine system
- Digestive system
- Urinary system
- Musculoskeletal system
- Integumentary system
- Immune system
- Lymphatic system
- Reproductive system
- Tips for studying anatomy and physiology

Box 7.2: Learning outcomes

By the end of this chapter, you should be able to

- Discuss the systems of the human body
- Understand how homeostasis works
- Define cells
- Identify the anatomy and physiology of the different systems of the human body
- Know how to write anatomy and physiology assignments.

DOI: 10.4324/9781003198338-10

Box 7.3: Keywords

- Anatomy
- Physiology
- Homeostasis
- Cells
- Oxygen (O_2)
- Carbon dioxide (CO_2)
- Systems
- Disease
- Heart
- Nervous system
- Digestive system
- Immune system
- Reproductive system
- Assignment writing

Box 7.4: Glossary

- Anatomy: position and structure of the body
- Physiology: function of the body
- Pathology: study of the cause and effect of a disease
- Pathophysiology: disordered physiological processes due to disease, injury or illness
- Homeostasis: maintenance of steady internal state despite internal and external variables

---

Introduction

A strong theoretical underpinning of anatomy, physiology and pathology is required to ensure that healthcare professionals and students have the skills and knowledge to provide effective care for patients in practice. This includes a comprehensive awareness of the key concepts of anatomy and physiology (A&P) in a healthy system and an understanding of the effects disease and illness have on the human body. It is impossible to cover A&P in the detail in this chapter. However, this chapter will introduce you to the key A&P concepts and give you the basic knowledge in preparation for further study on this topic.

This chapter will first describe the organisation of the body and then introduce the human systems and homeostasis, after which each system will then be discussed in detail. The final section of the chapter considers some tips for learners of A&P.

Organisation of the body

When studying A&P, it is useful to start with consideration of the organisation of the body. We tend to think of the human body as a whole (organism) or perhaps individual organs (heart, brain, skin, etc.). However, the human body can be split into six levels of structural organisation moving from the smallest structure to the human body as a whole.

- First level (chemical level): this is the first and smallest level of the structural hierarchy. This level involves atoms and the events occurring when atoms combine to form molecules
- Second level (cellular level): the next level is the cellular level. Cells are the smallest unit in all living things including humans, animals and plants. Cells will be looked in the subsequent sections
- Third level (tissue level): tissue is a structure in the human body made of two or more types of cells with a common function. There are four types of tissues in the human body:
  - Connective tissue: this tissue supports and binds body parts. Blood, cartilage and bone are examples of connective tissue
  - Epithelial tissue: this tissue lines and covers organs. Stomach and skin are lined with epithelial tissue
  - Muscle tissue: this tissue contracts and relaxes for movement of certain parts. Stomach, diaphragm and heart are all made of muscle tissue
  - Nervous tissue: this tissue senses stimuli and transmits impulses across the nervous system
- Fourth level (organ level): This structure is made of at least two different types of tissue to form an organ with specific function. The brain, heart and stomach are examples of organs
- Fifth level (organ system level): organ systems are one or more organs working together to perform a specific function. The digestive system, which includes the stomach, intestines and liver to digest and eliminate nutrients, is an example
- Sixth level (organism level): this is the largest level and includes all other organisational levels working together.

Activity 7.1: What are the common atoms and molecules?

An example of atoms and molecules most people are familiar with is 'H_2O', which is a combination of 2× hydrogen atoms and 1× oxygen atom.
  What are the common atoms and molecules listed below?

- C =
- H = Hydrogen
- = Oxygen
- CO_2 =

Cells

As explained previously, cells are the smallest unit that make up an organism. There are trillions of cells in the human body, and each cell type has a specific function in the body to ensure survival. They play a major role in protecting the body from pathogens (leucocytes), carrying oxygen to all parts of the body (erythrocytes) or forming part of the heart (cardiomyocytes). There are two broad categories of cells: eukaryotic and prokaryotic cells. Eukaryotic cells are those found in humans, animals and plants, whereas prokaryotic cells are found in bacteria. The simplest differentiation between the two broad categories is the inclusion of a membrane-bound nucleus, which is found in eukaryotic cells but not in prokaryotic cells. This section will focus on eukaryotic cells and will begin with the cell structure.

Cell structure

While each cell has a different function and role in the human body, almost all cells have a very similar structure. As mentioned above, eukaryotic cells are differentiated by their inclusion of a nucleus, which can be considered the 'brain' of the cell. This is one of the many organelles found in cellular structures ('organelle', much like an organ, refers to a specialised structure found in the cell). These organelles are held within the cell by a semi-permeable membrane and cytoplasm (Figure 7.1).

Nucleus

As noted earlier, the nucleus is considered the 'brain' or control centre of the cell. This is where the cells' genetic information (deoxyribonucleic acid [DNA]) is housed.

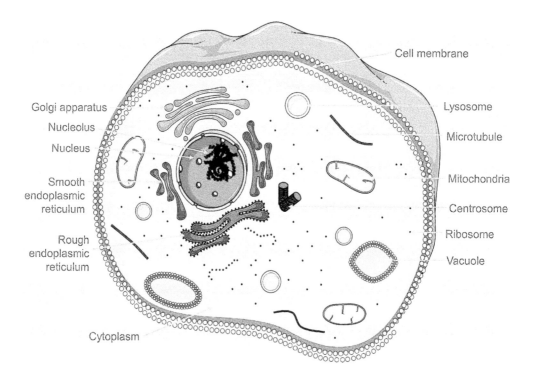

Figure 7.1 Cell structure
Creative Commons License

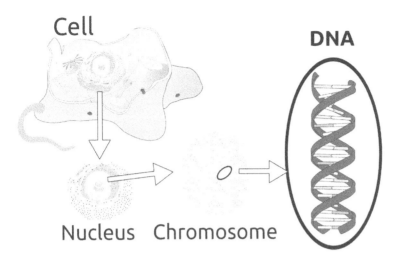

Figure 7.2 Nucleus
Creative Commons License

Table 7.1 Cellular organelles.

Ribosomes	Protein factories of the cell. They work with RNA codes to produce proteins
Mitochondria	Power house of the cell. Uses glucose to produce adenosine triphosphate, which is the energy source for the cell
Endoplasmic reticulum	Can be smooth or rough endoplasmic reticulum. Directs the movement of proteins and lipids
Golgi body	Processes and packages proteins and lipids to be removed from the cell
Lysosomes	'Rubbish collectors' of the cell, uses enzymes that break down unnecessary molecules and excretes or recycles them

DNA is the genetic blueprint of all cells and comprises four nitrogen-containing nucleobases: cytosine (C), guanine (G), thymine (T) and adenine (A). DNA provides instructions for ribonucleic acid (RNA), which transports this information out of the nucleus and (with the help of ribosomes, which is another organelle) then codes for various proteins.

DNA in the cell is housed in chromosomes present within the cell nucleus; each cell contains 46 chromosomes or 23 pairs, known as 'diploid cells'. These chromosomes are inherited from our parents, 23 pairs from the mother and 23 pairs from the father. Thus, sex cells (ova and sperm) are the only cells that are haploid, making 23 chromosomes in total.

Organelles

See Table 7.1 for a brief overview of some of the organelles found within cells.

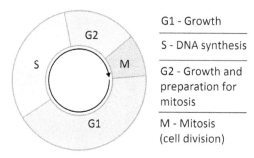

Figure 7.3 Cell cycle
Creative Commons License

Cell cycle

Most cells in the human body undergo cell division, a process wherein a cell divides and replicates into new cells. This process of cell division can be categorised as either mitosis or meiosis.

Mitosis refers to cell division seen in most of the cells within the human body. This is the process wherein cells divide into two *genetically identical daughter cells*. In cell cycle, the cell passes through different stages before division, including G1, S, G2 and M.

- G1 (growth): this is the stage wherein the cell begins preparing for mitosis S (DNA synthesis). DNA within the nucleus replicates to form two copies of DNA in preparation for cell division
- G2 (growth): this phase is another period of growth after DNA replication, again preparing for cell division. G1, S and G2 can also be referred to together as 'interphase'
- Mitosis (cell division): the cell divides into two identical daughter cells, and this process includes four main stages: prophase, metaphase, anaphase and telophase

The aim of mitosis is to ensure two genetically identical daughter cells are produced. However, it is possible for errors and mutations to occur during the interphase period. For example, during DNA synthesis, an error may indicate that not all chromosomes have split correctly. Throughout the cell cycle, checkpoints are in place in attempt to halt cell division should an error be noted. If, during this checkpoint, an error is noted, then the cell can attempt to rectify the error. If the error cannot be rectified, then this can result in apoptosis (cell death). These checkpoints are vitally important, as these errors in the cell cycle can develop into cancer.

'Meiosis' refers to cell division to produce gametes (ova or sperm cells). As mentioned above, sex cells contain only half the total number of chromosomes (23 chromosome in total). Meiosis results in four daughter cells as opposed to two identical daughter cells seen in mitosis. The process of meiosis begins similarly as mitosis, with the occurrence of DNA replication. However, the cells then go through two phases of mitosis (mitosis 1 and mitosis 2) to produce four haploid cells.

Different human systems and homeostasis

As described above, the human body can be split into various organ or body systems with specific structures and functions and that work together to maintain 'homeostasis'. What does this mean?

Homeostasis

'Homeostasis' refers to the maintenance of internal bodily conditions despite the constantly changing internal and external variables. For example, despite a range of external temperatures and physical activities, the human body will generally have a stable internal temperature of approximately 37 degrees Celsius. This process occurs through positive and negative feedback loops and specific feedback systems to maintain temperature control.

Feedback systems

Homeostatic feedback loops have three specific parts:

- Sensor: this includes receptors that detect a physiological value
- Control centre: it receives information from the sensor and interprets the value in comparison to the set parameters and prepares a response
- Effector: this receives information from the control centre and initiates change to restore balance

Using temperature as an example:

- Sensor: peripheral temperature increases past set point owing to hot external weather or physical activity
- Control centre: The thermoregulatory centre of the brain receives this information and interprets that temperature has increased above set point and that the temperature needs to be lowered
- Effector: vasodilation occurs within blood vessels to increase heat loss (skin appears flushed), and sweat glands secrete fluids, which cool the temperature by evaporation. This lowers down the overall body temperature to the set parameters (37 degrees Celsius)

Temperature control is a good example of homeostatic control and balance; however, homeostatic control refers to a huge variety of body processes including blood glucose control, blood CO_2/O_2 control, blood clotting and water balance.

Homeostatic control follows two set feedback loops, namely, negative and positive feedback loops:

- Negative feedback loop: this is the most common feedback loop in the human body. It aims to ensure maintenance of certain parameters (that is, temperature control) and to adjust responses accordingly to restore the set parameters. This feedback loop is also seen in blood glucose control and water balance

- Positive feedback loop: this loop works to increase the imbalance in the change. For example, this feedback is seen in blood clotting: a tear in a blood vessel causes platelets (blood cells responsible for blood clotting) to adhere to the tear and release chemicals that attract more platelets, which, in turn, release more chemicals, and so on

Homeostatic imbalance can be the cause or consequence of many diseases. For example, type 1 diabetes causes a homeostatic imbalance of blood glucose control as insulin-producing cells are destroyed, resulting in blood sugar control being inefficient to maintain homeostatic control.

We will now look at each of these systems in detail.

Nervous system

Primary function (physiology)

The nervous system is the body's primary command centre, as it collects information from both the internal and external environments, interprets this information and responds accordingly. It is also in control of what makes you… you! It creates thoughts, remembers past events and is responsible for behaviours and personality.

Structure (anatomy)

The nervous system can be divided into two main parts: central nervous system (CNS) and peripheral nervous system (PNS). The CNS comprises the brain and spinal cord. The PNS consists of nerves and supporting nervous system cells (neuroglial cells) outside of the brain and spinal cord.

PNS can be further divided into:

- Somatic nervous system: it regulates activities under conscious or voluntary control, that is, muscle and skeletal movements for walking
- Autonomic nervous system: it regulates activities under unconscious or involuntary control, that is, heart rate and digestion. The autonomic nervous system can be further subdivided into
  - Sympathetic nervous system (the fight or flight response): this involuntarily prepares the body for stress-related activities by rapidly changing physiological processes within the body, such as by increasing heart rate, blood pressure and pupil dilation and reducing digestion
  - Parasympathetic nervous system (the rest and digest response): this is responsible for involuntary day-to-day physiological processes in the human body. It is also responsible for the stimulation of the digestive and urinary systems, reduction of heart rate and blood pressure and constriction of pupil dilation

Neurons

A neuron is one of the primary cells that make up the nervous system, including the CNS and PNS. Neurons communicate through chemical and electrical signals, whereby they receive information from neighbouring cells in the internal environment or information

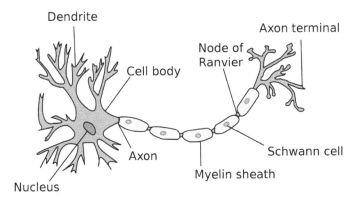

Figure 7.4 Neurons
Creative Commons License

from the external environment and transmit this information through the PNS to the CNS for interpretation by the brain and transmit responses back to the PNS through the spinal cord.

Neurons differ from other eukaryotic cells in structure for an enhance rapid transfer of information across the nervous system and include two specialised structures seen only in neurons: dendrites and axon.

Dendrites are extensions of the neuron that branch out from the cell body and receive and process incoming signals from the surrounding environment.

An axon is a single fibre that carries the message away from the cell body towards the next neuron. Axons are often covered with a fatty substance called myeline sheath, which protects the axon and helps speed up information transfer.

Neuroglia

Neurons are responsible for information transfer in the nervous system, and neuroglia (also known as glial cells) make up the numerous specialised cells also seen within the nervous system. The neuroglial cells are responsible for supporting, protecting and maintaining the nervous system and neurons. These cells include microglia, which provides immune support for the CNS, and Schwann cells and oligodendrocytes, which form the myelin sheath in the PNS and CNS, respectively.

Cardiovascular system

Primary function (physiology)

The function of the cardiovascular system (CVS) is to maintain a continuous blood flow to all body cells to ensure an adequate supply of oxygen and other nutrients to maintain homeostasis and ensure optimum body functioning. The CVS is an effective transport system that works closely with the respiratory system to support the body's necessary functions.

Structure (anatomy)

The CVS has two main parts:

- The heart: a muscular pump that circulates blood continuously throughout the body
- Blood vessels: the circulatory system forms a network of vessels around the body, named blood vessels, through which the blood flows

---

Activity 7.2: Structures of the cardiovascular system

Spend a few moments writing down as many structures of the cardiovascular system that you can think of. Think about different parts of the heart and blood vessels that you may have come across previously.

How did you do in Activity 7.2? Could you name any valves or chambers of the heart, or any major blood vessels? You might have referred to, for example, atrium, ventricle, aorta, pulmonary artery, pulmonary vein, superior and inferior vena cava, pulmonary valve, tricuspid valve, bicuspid valve, aortic valve, myocardium, pericardium and septum.

The heart

The heart is a muscular organ located between the lungs in the thoracic cavity, in an area known as the mediastinum, which is present slightly towards the left. It is cone-shaped and nearly the size of your fist and has four chambers. Each day, it pumps approximately 5 litres of blood throughout the body.

The wall of the heart has three layers:

- Pericardium: this is the outer layer that has two sacs: the outer sac, made of fibrous tissue, and the inner sac, made of a double-layered serous membrane
- Myocardium: this is the middle layer and is made of specialised cardiac muscle, and it is found only within the heart. Within the myocardium is a network of specialised cells responsible for transmitting the heart's electrical signals
- Endocardium: this is the innermost layer and lines the heart's chambers and valves. It's a thin, smooth membrane that facilitates the blood flow throughout the heart

Blood supply to the heart (coronary circulation)

Arterial blood flow to the heart is facilitated by the coronary arteries, which are the branches of the aorta forming a vast network of capillaries that supply blood to the heart, especially the muscle of the left ventricle. The latter is responsible for pumping the blood around the body, initially through the aorta.

Venous drainage from the heart occurs through the cardiac veins.

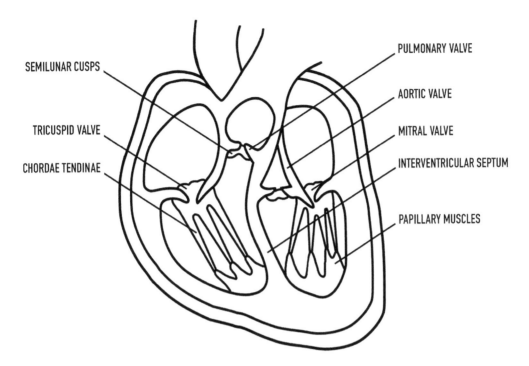

PULMONARY VALVE

AORTIC VALVE

MITRAL VALVE

INTERVENTRICULAR SEPTUM

PAPILLARY MUSCLES

SEMILUNAR CUSPS

TRICUSPID VALVE

CHORDAE TENDINAE

Figure 7.5 Heart
Image credit: Tamsin Arai Drake

The chambers of the heart

The heart has two upper chambers, known as atria, and two lower chambers, known as ventricles. Following birth, the heart is divided into the right and left sides, separated by the septum, and the blood cannot cross the septum.

Valves of the heart

The atria and ventricles present on each side of the heart are divided by an atrio-ventricular (AV) valve, which, on the right side of the heart, is known as the tri-cuspid valve and, on the left side, the mitral valve. This value has two cusp or flaps. The chordae tendineae prevent these valves from opening in the upwards direction towards the atria.

The pulmonary valve is located at the entrance to the pulmonary artery, and the aortic valve is located at the entrance to the aorta to prevent backflow of blood when the ventricular muscles relax.

Blood flow through the heart

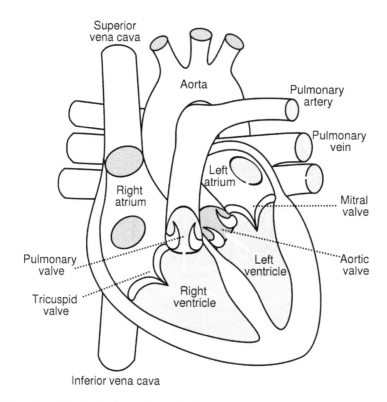

Figure 7.6 Blood circulation through the heart
Creative Commons License

Conduction pathway of the heart

The heart generates its own electrical impulses, which initiate the heartbeat. The pathway for the heart's beating mechanism includes five elements:

- Sinoatrial (SA) node: this is called the pacemaker of the heart and is found in the wall of the right atrium, and firing of the SA node triggers the atria to contract
- AV node: this is found in the wall of the atrial septum near the AV valves and transmits the signal from the atria to ventricles
- The bundle of His: this is a mass of specialised fibres that begin contraction of the ventricles
- Left and right bundle branches: these are further branched structures of specialised fibres
- The Purkinje conductivity fibres: the bundle of His, bundle branches and Purkinje fibres transmit electrical impulses from the AV node to the myocardium, causing ventricular contraction and resulting in pumping of blood into the aorta and pulmonary artery

The cardiac cycle

The cardiac cycle involves the following phases:

- Contraction: systole
- Relaxation: diastole
- Depolarization: release of electrical stimulus
- Repolarization: recharge phase

Cardiac output is a measure of the heart's efficiency. It is calculated by the heart rate (that is, the number of times the heart beats per minute and the stroke volume – the amount of blood ejected in millilitres each time the heart beats).

Blood vessels and the circulatory system

To understand the circulatory system, it is best viewed as two distinctive parts, although these parts work continuously together to circulate blood around the body. The parts are:

- Pulmonary circulation (heart and lungs)
- Systemic circulation (body or general circulation)

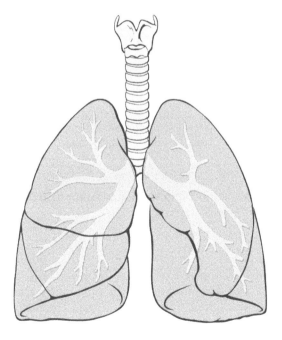

Figure 7.7 Lungs
Creative Commons License

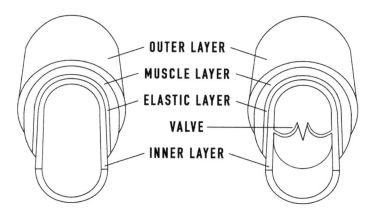

Figure 7.8 Blood vessels
Image credit: Tamsin Arai Drake

Panel 7.1: Lung function

The pulmonary circulation (involving the heart and lungs)

- Carries DEOXYGENATED blood away from the RIGHT VENTRICLE of the heart to the lungs
- Returns OXYGENATED blood to the LEFT ATRIUM

The systemic circulation (involving the body)

- Carries OXYGENATED BLOOD away from the LEFT VENTRICLE
- Supplies oxygenated blood to the body tissues
- Returns DEOXYGENATED BLOOD from the body tissues
- Takes it back to the RIGHT ATRIUM

The circulatory system is made of a network of blood vessels comprising the arteries and veins of varying sizes. The walls of all blood vessels have three layers.

Arteries

Arteries generally carry oxygenated blood at high pressure away from the heart and have a thicker muscle layer in the vessel wall (the exception is the pulmonary artery, which carries deoxygenated blood from the right atrium to the lungs). The aorta is the largest artery in the body, which carries oxygenated blood from the left ventricle to the entire body. The arteries then branch out into smaller vessels called arterioles, which further divide into capillaries. Capillaries have a thin cell wall that allows exchange of substances between the blood and body tissues across a semi-permeable cell membrane.

Other arteries in the body include those in the head and neck (left and right carotid, external carotid and vertebral), those in the torso (bronchial, oesophageal, intercostal and pericardial) and those in the abdomen (inferior and superior mesenteric, renal, lumbar and common iliac). There are also arteries in the arms and legs.

Veins

Veins generally carry deoxygenated blood at lower pressure and have thinner vessel walls and valves to prevent backflow (the exception is the pulmonary veins, which return oxygenated blood from the lungs to the left atrium). The two largest veins in the body are the superior and inferior vena cava, which return deoxygenated blood from the entire body to the right atrium of the heart. Veins ae also subdivided into smaller vessels called venules.

Other veins in the body include those in the head and neck, torso and upper and lower extremities.

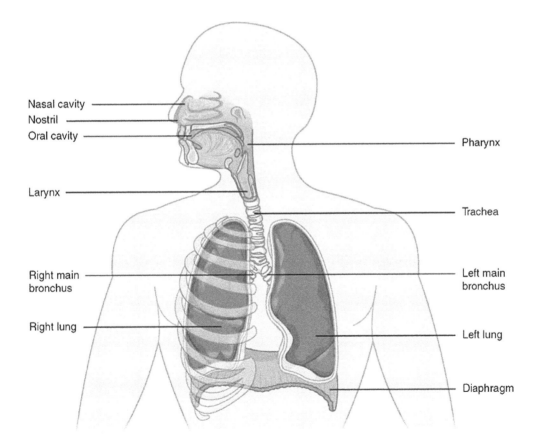

Figure 7.9 Respiratory organs
Creative Commons License

Respiratory system

Primary function (physiology)

The respiratory system's primary function is to facilitate gas exchange, by taking up oxygen (O_2) from the environment and carrying it throughout the body via the bloodstream to be used in cellular respiration. This system also removes a by-product of cellular respiration, namely, carbon dioxide (CO_2).

Structure (anatomy)

The respiratory system can be broadly divided into the upper and lower respiratory tracts. The upper respiratory tract comprises the nose, pharynx and larynx, whereas the lower respiratory tract includes the trachea, lungs and diaphragm.

The upper respiratory tract is responsible for the inhalation of environmental air. As environmental air is taken up through the upper respiratory tract and moves towards the lower respiratory tract, where it is warmed, moistened and filtered.

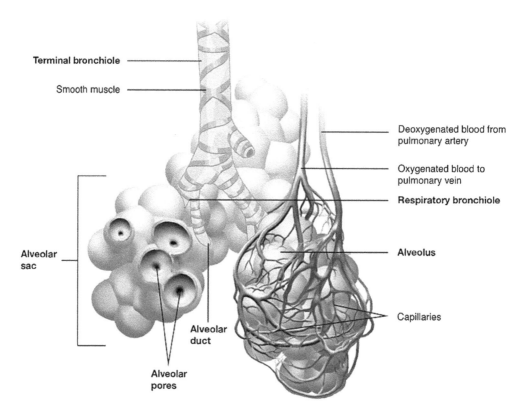

Figure 7.10 Respiratory zone

Once the air reaches the trachea (also known as the windpipe), it has entered the lower respiratory tract. The movement of air through the respiratory tract is achieved by ventilation (the physical act of breathing), contraction/relaxation of muscles surrounding the lungs and the pulling in and pushing out of air by the diaphragm.

Once the air reaches the lung, it passes down through smaller structures within the lung—bronchi → bronchioles → alveoli sac → alveoli. As mentioned earlier, the primary function of the respiratory system is to facilitate the process of gas exchange (also referred to as respiration), and this process occurs within the alveoli in the lungs through the process of diffusion (the movement of molecules from an area of high concentration to that of low concentration).

Gas exchange

Cells require O_2 as part of their cellular metabolism (energy for the cell) and need a near-constant supply. O_2 in inspired air diffuses across the alveoli wall into deoxygenated blood supplied by the CVS. The oxygenated blood then moves around the body through the CVS where the O_2 again diffuses across cell walls to be used within the cell. The by-product, CO_2, also moves from the cell to the bloodstream and is carried by the CVS to the alveoli, where it is exhaled. This is the process of gas exchange and can also be referred to as external respiration (movement of O_2/CO_2 in the alveoli) and internal respiration (movement of O_2/CO_2 within the cells).

Endocrine system

Primary function (physiology)

The endocrine system works closely with the nervous system and CVS to co-ordinate the body's activities and maintain homeostasis. Where the nervous system can create a

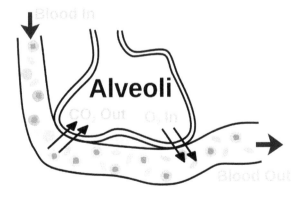

Figure 7.11 Gas exchange
Creative Commons License

rapid change, the endocrine system has a slower effect, but its actions usually last longer. The primary function of the endocrine system is to release hormones and to maintain the appropriate level of hormones needed by the body systems. It carries out these functions in conjunction with the nervous system through feedback mechanisms.

Endocrine hormones are chemical messengers that act mostly by attaching to specific receptors on the cell membrane to deliver their signals.

Structure (anatomy)

The endocrine system comprises a collection of glands, distributed throughout the body but not physically connected to each other, and the glands produce hormones.

The pituitary gland is known as the 'master gland', as it secretes primary hormones that influence the release of secondary hormones from other glands. It works closely with the hypothalamus (the key integrating link between the nervous and endocrine systems)

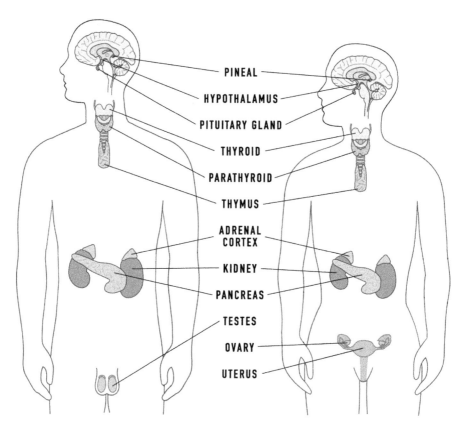

Figure 7.12 Endocrine system
Image credit: Tamsin Arai Drake,
adapted from: Creative Commons License

to maintain homeostasis by acting on the messages received through feedback systems. Together the hypothalamus and pituitary play important roles in most aspects of growth, development and metabolism.

The anterior pituitary gland secretes:

- Adrenocorticotrophic hormone: this stimulates the adrenal glands to produce hormones
- Thyroid-stimulating hormone: this stimulates the thyroid gland to produce hormones
- Luteinising hormone (LH): this stimulates the development of testes and ovaries
- Follicle-stimulating hormone (FSH): this stimulates the development of follicles
- Prolactin: this stimulates mammary gland growth and milk production
- Growth hormone: this stimulates muscle and skeletal growth and stimulates the liver to produce growth factors that stimulate bone and cartilage growth
- Melanocyte-stimulating hormone: this influences pigmentation of the skin, hair and eyes

The posterior pituitary gland secretes antidiuretic hormone, which stimulates the retention of water and oxytocin, causing uterine contractions and milk ejection reflex in the mammary glands.

Other endocrine glands are:

- Pineal gland: this releases melatonin and is involved in daily and seasonal rhythmic activities/sleep patterns, regulated by light/dark
- Thyroid gland: this produces T3 (triiodothyronine) and T4 (thyroxine) from the thyroid follicles, wherein iodine atoms are attaching to tyrosine. T3 and T4 affect most of the cells in the body, thereby increasing the basal metabolic rate and heat production and regulating the metabolism of carbohydrates, fats and proteins. These hormones are essential for normal growth and development. The gland also produces calcitonin, which lowers calcium levels in the body by promoting the storage of calcium in the bones and inhibiting the reabsorption of calcium by the kidneys.
- Parathyroid gland: this gland works in partnership with calcitonin produced from the thyroid gland to maintain levels of blood calcium. Calcium levels influence muscle contraction, nerve transmission and blood clotting
- Thymus gland: this gland plays a significant role in supporting immune system immunity by producing thymosin, which stimulates the development of T-lymphocytes (T cells–white blood cells [WBCs])
- Adrenal glands: the adrenal cortex produces hormones that control sex (testosterone and oestrogen) and sodium balance in the blood (aldosterone), which affects blood pressure and glucose balance (cortisol). The adrenal medulla produces hormones involved in the fight-or-flight response (adrenaline and noradrenaline)
- Kidneys: They secrete hormones such as the those of the renin–angiotensin system, which controls blood pressure, and erythropoietin, which controls red blood cell production (erythropoiesis), and the final activation of vitamin D to the active hormone calcitriol occurs in the kidneys

- Pancreas: Its endocrine function is to regulate blood glucose levels.

    Two main pancreatic hormones produced by the Islets of Langerhans are

    Insulin produced by beta cells, which lowers elevated blood glucose levels; and glucagon, produced by alpha cells, which increase blood glucose concentrations from inadequate levels
- Testes: These produce testosterone, which regulates sperm production
- Ovaries: These produce the female sex hormones oestrogen and progesterone, which regulate the female reproductive cycle, thus maintaining pregnancy and preparing mammary glands for lactation. Ovaries also produce relaxin, which inhibits uterine smooth muscle contraction and dilates the cervix during labour, and inhibin, which inhibits the release of FSH

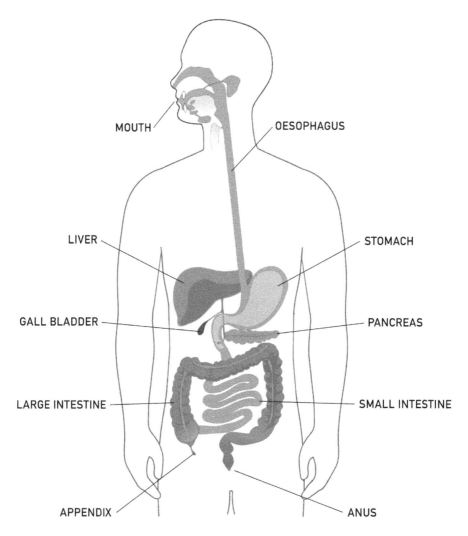

Figure 7.13 Digestive system
Image Credit: Tamsin Arai, adapted from: Creative Commons License

Endocrine hormones enter the blood stream, wherein they circulate and target not only cells distant from the glands that secrete them but also cells that have receptors that can specifically bind hormones.

Digestive system

Primary function (physiology)

All processes within the human body require energy, which we receive through food and fluids. The digestive system's primary task is to convert dietary intake into nutrients and energy, which is used by our cells and body systems for all functions. The digestive system breaks down, absorbs and eliminates waste products with the aid of specific digestive organs and accessory organs.

Structure (anatomy)

The structure of the digestive system can be divided into the gastrointestinal (GI) tract (also referred to as the alimentary canal) and accessory organs.

Gastrointestinal tract

The GI tract is a hollow tube beginning from the mouth, which then passes down through the hollow organs including the oesophagus, stomach, small intestines, large intestines and the anus. Food and fluid pass through the GI tract, where they undergo the process of ingestion, digestion, absorption and elimination with the assistance of the digestive accessory organs, the liver, gallbladder and pancreas.

Activity 7.3: Chemical/mechanical digestion

Digestion occurs in the body by either mechanical or chemical digestion. This is the method by which food is broken down within the gastrointestinal tract.

- Mechanical digestion is the physical movement that causes the breakdown of food
- Chemical digestion relates to the liquids and enzymes causing the breakdown of food
- Mechanical and chemical digestion occurs in most parts of the gastrointestinal tract. For example, food is chewed within the mouth and then coated with saliva before being swallowed. Chewing is the first stage of mechanical breakdown, and saliva contains enzymes that begin the chemical breakdown of our food.

Can you think of what other forms of mechanical/chemical breakdown occur within the GI tract? Consider what is happening in the stomach and intestines.

The accessory organs comprising part of the GI tract are not hollow organs. They do not come into contact with the ingested material within the GI tract and can be seen as having a supporting role within the digestive tract. Their role revolves around aiding chemical digestion through bile or enzyme production, which is introduced into the small intestine.

Ingestion

The first stage in the digestive system is simply the ingestion of food/fluids into the body normally through the mouth, where food is chewed and coated with saliva before being passed through the pharynx into the oesophagus. Generally, the food we eat cannot be absorbed into the body and used as energy in the intact form, and the main function of the digestive system is to break food into small parts that can be absorbed and used. This is why digestion is one of the most drawn-out processes of the digestive system and occurs through most parts of the GI tract.

Digestion

To break down the food you have just eaten, a series of chemical and mechanical methods of digestion occur throughout the body. This occurs primarily through the mouth, stomach and small intestine: turning a cheeseburger, for example, into fats, carbohydrates, minerals and vitamins, all of which the body can absorb and use as building blocks. Accessory organs of the digestive system assist in the chemical digestion of food, with bile produced in the liver and stored in the gallbladder breaking down fats and lipids. Pancreatic enzymes are released by the exocrine pancreas into the small intestine assisting in the breakdown of fats, carbohydrates, proteins and peptides.

Once these molecules are degraded into small particles, they can then be absorbed through the semi-permeable digestive membrane into the blood and transported around the body for use or storage. This primarily occurs within the small intestine. Once food (referred to as 'chyme' after it passes through the stomach and then into the small intestine) enters the large intestine, much of the absorption has occurred, and the remaining product is prepared for elimination, which is known as faeces. Faeces contain a mixture of undigested food, live and dead bacteria, cells and digestive secretions such as bile.

Urinary system

Primary function (physiology)

The urinary system's primary function is to excrete waste products produced by the body. It does this by filtering the blood and excreting wasting products through urine. It also plays a role in controlling blood pressure, balancing fluid levels and maintaining homeostasis.

Structure (anatomy)

The urinary system consists of two kidneys (right and left), ureter, bladder and urethra. The processes of filtration and absorption occur within the kidneys where urine is

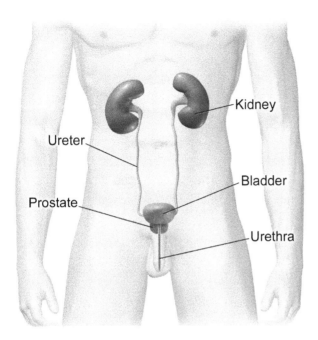

Figure 7.14 Urinary system
Creative Commons License

generated, which is then passed down the ureter, stored in the bladder and expelled through the urethra.

The kidneys

Most of the work of the urinary system is done within the kidneys. The renal artery supplies blood to the kidneys, where filtration occurs, and is then carried away by the renal vein. Blood is passed through a structure called a 'nephron'. A nephron is the kidney's filtering unit, and there are approximately one million nephrons in each kidney.

The key structures to be aware of within a nephron are the glomerulus (encased by Bowman's capsule), proximal convoluted tubule (PCT), loop of Henle and distal convoluted tubule (DCT).

Blood enters the glomerulus and passes plasma into the Bowman's capsule through a semi-permeable membrane. Once this liquid enters the Bowman's capsule, it is referred to as 'filtrate' and contains molecules such as urea, creatine, glucose and amino acids. The filtrate is then passed through the PCT, loop of Henle and DCT. During this time, important molecules (such as glucose) and water are reabsorbed back into the bloodstream. Remaining waste products (such as urea) are passed on to the collecting duct into the ureter and expelled as urine.

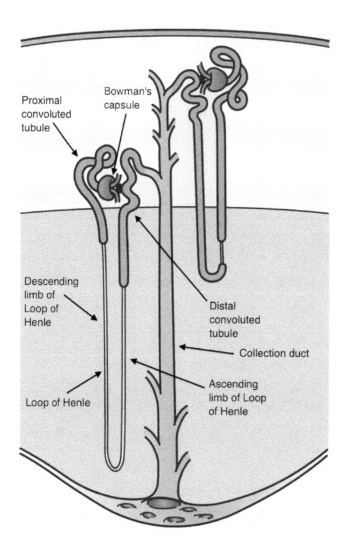

Figure 7.15 Nephron
Creative Commons License

Urination (micturition)

Urine is the end product of filtration and reabsorption of filtrate within the nephrons. Once formed, urine is passed into the ureters and stored in the bladder. As the bladder fills, pressure sensors send signals to the brain to indicate the need for urination. The external urethral sphincter is under conscious control and allows urination to occur at the right time (unless there is some form of urinary incontinence), allowing urine to pass through the urethra and expel from the body.

Musculoskeletal system

Primary function (physiology)

The musculoskeletal (MSK) system consists of the bones and soft tissues—tendons, ligaments, cartilage and muscles—which provide a framework for the body, allowing movement, posture and body weight balance.

Structure (anatomy)

MSK system provides a framework to the human skeleton, with the associated soft tissues (muscles, tendons, etc.) creating the MSK system. The human skeleton has 206 bones, which provide this framework, ranging in size and function. Bones provide protection for internal structures, for example, the rib cage protects the heart and lungs. Bones also provide strength and movement, with the pelvis supporting the upper body and allowing movement through the hips and legs.

Bones

Bones are a connective tissue that make up the human skeleton. The skeleton can be divided into two broad categories: axial and appendicular skeleton.

Panel 7.2: Human skeleton

The axial skeleton includes the skull, ribs and vertebra and provides support and movement as well as protects internal organs such as the brain, heart and lungs.

   The appendicular skeleton includes all other bones that are attached to the axial skeleton, such as the femur (thigh bone), and its primary function is to enable movement.

Within the skeleton, there are five different types of bones:

- Long bones: for movement and support, present in the arms and legs (radius and femur)
- Short bones: these provide stability and movement, present in the wrists and ankles (carpels and tarsals)
- Flat bones: these protect internal organs such as the brain and heart (skull and ribs)
- Irregular bones: these aid in load bearing and protection, present in the spine (vertebra)
- Sesamoid bones: These increase weight bearing and tolerance by supporting tendons, present in the knee (patella)

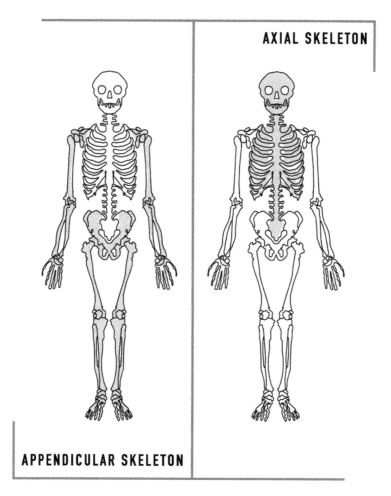

Figure 7.16 Skeletal system
Image credit: Tamsin Arai Drake

Joints

Movement is an important function of the MSK system, and the ability to move depends on the connection of these bones within the skeletal system. These connections are called joints, and they occur where two or more bones join. Joints vary within the skeleton and are classified depending on the amount of movement they permit.

- Fibrous joints: usually offer no movement
- Cartilaginous joints: offer minimal movement
- Synovial joints: offer a range of movements. Synovial joints are further categorised depending on the type of movement needed

Bones are attached to connecting bones by ligaments. Ligaments provide support and stability during movement while also preventing movement in the wrong direction.

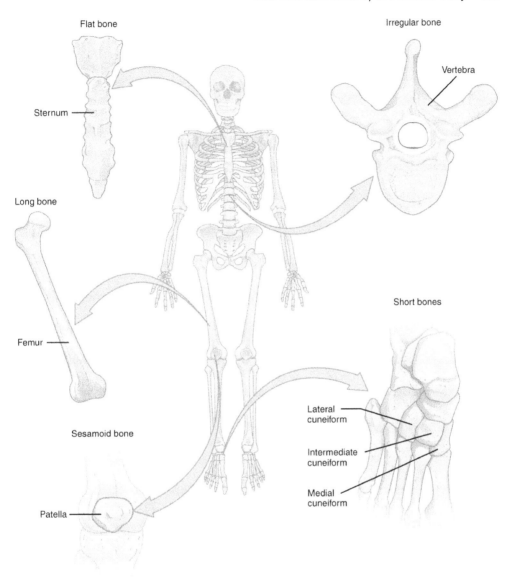

Flat bone

Irregular bone

Vertebra

Sternum

Long bone

Femur

Short bones

Sesamoid bone

Lateral cuneiform

Intermediate cuneiform

Medial cuneiform

Patella

Figure 7.17 Bone classification
Creative Commons License

Skeletal muscle

With all muscles, the key characteristic of the skeletal muscle is the ability to relax and contract, which causes movement. Skeletal muscles are connected to bones through tendons, and their contraction and relaxation pull the associated bone, which causes movement. This movement is under voluntary control and is one of the differences between other muscle types (cardiac/smooth muscle is under unconscious/involuntary control).

Integumentary system

Primary function (physiology)

The integumentary system contains the largest organ in the human body (the skin), and its primary function is to form a physical barrier from the outside world, protecting the internal environment from external factors. It also has a role in other functions such as fluid balance, temperature regulation and vitamin synthesis and contains nerve endings responsible for the detection of stimuli (pain, touch, pressure, etc.).

Structure (anatomy)

The integumentary system includes the skin, which can be divided into epidermis, dermis and subcutaneous tissue (hypodermis) and includes glands, nails and hair.

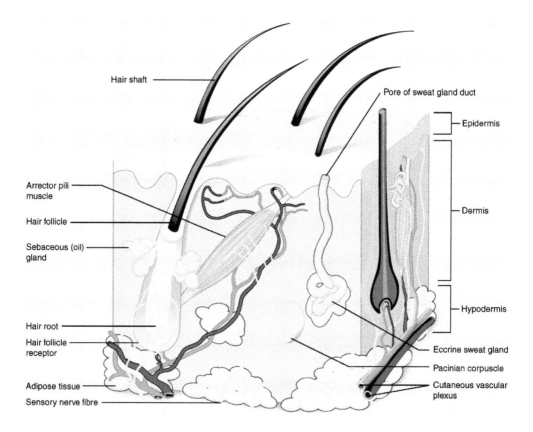

Figure 7.18 Structure of the skin
Creative Commons License

The skin

As already mentioned, the skin can be split into three main sections:

- Epidermis: this is the outermost layer of the skin and the layer that is the part you can see with the naked eye. The epidermis is strong, resilient and elastic. While the epidermis is visible to the naked eye, the fact that the epidermis is arranged as a layer-by-layer of cells is not visible. Lacking blood supply, nutrients are received from the underlying dermis and do not reach the cells in the outer layer of the epidermis. This causes these cells to die and shed as they reach the outermost layers; they are thus continually being replaced by the underlying cells
- Dermis: this is the underlying structure below the epidermis and is a connective tissue framework. The dermis consists of two separate layers: the papillary region, which lies below the epidermis, and the reticular region, which is the second layer of the dermis and lies above the hypodermis. The dermis contains blood, lymph vessels, sweat glands, nerves and hair follicles
- Hypodermis: this layer lies below the dermis and above the underlying structures and consists of connective tissue and fatty tissue (adipose tissue). The hypodermis plays an important role in temperature control and energy storage.

Immune system

Primary function (physiology)

The immune system's primary function is to protect us from potential infection and limit infection if a pathogen (disease-causing agent) enters the body. It primarily comprises immune cells (WBCs) produced in the bone marrow and includes proteins and organs that help protect the human body.

Structure (anatomy)

The immune system comprises trillions of cells that aid in the protection of the body. Produced in the bone marrow, immune cells are carried through the bloodstream and lymphatic fluid and housed in the lymph nodes. The immune system can be categorised into two lines of defence: innate and adaptive immune systems.

Innate and adaptive immune systems

The innate immune system is the body's immune system present from birth and responds quickly to protect the body. This can also be referred to as the non-specific immune system. The innate immune system comprises defence mechanisms such as the skin, stomach acid, inflammatory response and specific WBCs (see Table 7.2).

Inflammatory response

The inflammatory response is a key part of the body's non-specific (innate) immune system, and everyone has encountered such a response at some point in their lives. The inflammatory response is a straightforward mode by which the body responds to injury or infection, thus producing pain, swelling and heat in the affected area (for example, a

Table 7.2 Innate and adaptive immune systems.

Cell	Function	Innate/adaptive
Neutrophil	One of the first cells to respond to invading microbes and destroys microbes by ingesting them (phagocytosis)	Innate
Macrophage	Phagocytises microbes, releases molecules to stimulate inflammation/immune response and works with T cells by presenting antigens	Innate
Natural killer cell	Destroys infected cells by injecting a protein that causes apoptosis (cell death). This can be cells infected with viruses or cancerous cells	Innate
B lymphocyte (B cell)	Antibody-producing cells; antibodies attach to specific bacteria and viruses (antigens) and neutralise them	Adaptive
T lymphocyte (T cell)	Attacks microbes directly and works together with macrophage cells to be spoon-fed cells	Adaptive

scratch on your hand). Because of the injury/infection, damaged cells release chemicals that initiate the inflammatory response, causing WBCs to rush to the site to clear up any possible microbes and begin the healing process.

Systemic fever is another sign of the body's innate inflammatory response. If the body recognises a pathogenic infection (that is, bacterial or viral infection), then the hypothalamus increases the body temperature beyond 38 degrees Celsius to kill the pathogen, which cannot survive at higher temperatures.

Adaptive immune system

The adaptive immune system comprises the body's specific immune response. If the body's innate immune system is overrun and cannot eliminate the pathogen, then our body's adaptive immune system can assist. However, this immune system provides a slow response to infection and takes time to develop an immune response to a specific pathogen. Lymphocytes (T cells and B cells) react only to specific pathogens they are 'trained' to fight with after an initial exposure. The adaptive immune system is the reason why, as children, we are generally more unwell with viruses such as common cold. However, as we age and encounter these viruses again, our adaptive immune system 'remembers' these viruses and can respond quickly and neutralise them before we become unwell. This results in naturally acquired immunity.

The adaptive immune system can become naturally immune to pathogens due to previous exposure (that is, common cold and chicken pox). However, this immunity can also be artificially acquired; a good example of this is vaccination. Vaccinations provide an initial immune response to a specific disease, which means that if a person is exposed to the same disease later, the adaptive immune system can produce an immune response and prevent illness or severe illness.

Lymphatic system

Primary function (physiology)

The lymphatic system works closely with both the immune system and the CVS, assisting in the storage and movement of WBCs and 'mopping up' excess fluid from tissues and returning it back to the bloodstream. The fluid transported around the lymphatic system is referred to as 'lymph' and is a clear colourless liquid.

Structure (anatomy)

The lymphatic system's structure centres around a series of lymphatic vessels, lymphatic ducts and lymph nodes to transport lymph around the body. The structure of the lymphatic system resembles that of the CVS, with smaller lymphatic capillaries feeding into bigger vessels and ducts towards the heart, which is then returned to the venous system for recirculation. Unlike the CVS, the lymphatic system is a pumpless system and depends on muscle contraction and surrounding movement (cardiovascular arteries pulsating and physical movement) to push the lymph fluid through the lymphatic system.

The lymph is passed through different nodes situated throughout the lymphatic system. Lymph nodes are situated throughout the lymphatic system but are found in clusters around the mouth, groin, armpit, digestive system and pharynx. Lymph nodes can be thought of as filters or checkpoints throughout the body, filtering and checking the lymph

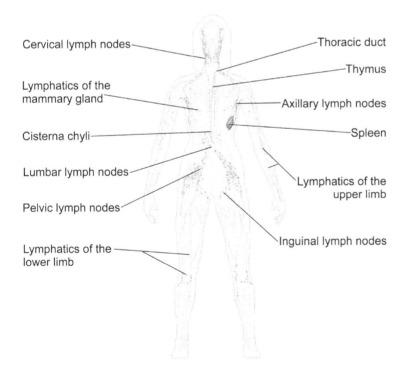

Figure 7.19 Lymphatic system

fluid for signs of infection. Lymphocytes (WBCs) are housed within the lymph nodes and assist in clearing out potential infections (pathogens) if found within the lymph node. Owing to its filtration function, lymph nodes can become overwhelmed if systemic infection is present, resulting in swollen, painful lymph nodes.

Reproductive system

Primary function (physiology)

The reproductive system is unique in the human body, as it is the only system with clear differences between male and female biology. However, the primary function remains the same and revolves around continuation of the species.

Through the menstrual cycle in females and sperm production in males, the reproductive system works to ensure fertilisation can occur. The female reproductive system ensures that gestation of a foetus, and delivery and nurturing of the new-born, takes place. More information regarding reproductive hormones can be found in the endocrine section of this chapter.

Structure (anatomy)

The male reproductive system includes the testes, prostate gland and penis. Within this structure, sperm are continually produced, matured and stored, ready for delivery to the female reproductive system. The primary male sex hormone testosterone is synthesised within the testes and is responsible for the development of male characteristics and structures such as testes, body hair and changes to muscle mass.

The female reproductive system contains internal structures such as the ovaries, fallopian tubes, uterus and vagina and external structures of the vulva, such as the labia majora, labia minora and clitoris and the breasts. Unlike the male reproductive system, females are born with all of the egg cells (ova) required within their lifetime, and these are stored within the ovaries ready for release and fertilisation with the sperm. The main female sex hormones are released by the ovaries and fluctuate in amount depending on the menstrual cycle.

The menstrual cycle

The menstrual cycle is a monthly cycle that results in normal hormonal and structural changes within the female reproductive system to make pregnancy possible. This includes both an ovarian cycle and a uterine cycle, which occur concurrently. On average, a menstrual cycle can occur between 20 and 35 days; however, for this chapter, we will assume a 28-day cycle, with day 1 being the first day of menses (first day of bleeding).

Ovarian cycle

The ovarian cycle describes the period of maturation of follicles (immature egg cells; also referred to as 'oocyte') already present within the ovary and can be divided into three stages: follicular phase, ovulation phase and luteal phase.

The first stage in the ovarian cycle begins on day 1 of menses (day 1/28) and continues until mid-cycle (day 14). This period is characterised with high levels of FSH that stimulates the development of follicles within the ovary in preparation for ovulation. When levels of FSH (and LH) peak, it triggers the eruption of the oocyte. The oocyte then travels along the fallopian tube ready to be fertilised. From days 15 to 24, the ovarian cycle focuses on the development of the corpus luteum—a collection of cells within the ovary. The eruption of the oocyte leads to the development of the corpus luteum within the ovary. The corpus luteum releases progesterone, which prepares the uterus for pregnancy. If left unfertilised, the corpus luteum degenerates before the next cycle, where the cycle then repeats.

The uterine cycle

During the ovarian cycle, the uterus also undergoes changes in preparation for a fertilised egg cell to implant itself into its wall. It can also be split into three phases: menses, proliferative and secretory phase. Menstruation occurs between days 1 and 5 of the uterine cycle. When no fertilised egg is implanted into the uterine wall during the last cycle, the uterine lining (also referred to as endometrium) sheds in preparation for the next uterine layer to form. This 'old' blood and tissue is then expelled through the cervix and vagina, resulting in a period. During days 6–14 of the cycle, high levels of oestrogen cause fresh tissue to grow within the womb, and this also includes developing an increased blood supply within the tissue. This tissue will house and nourish a fertilised egg in the early stages of pregnancy once it is implanted in the uterine wall. Progesterone released by the corpus luteum further thickens the endometrium during days 15–28 of the cycle. If no fertilised egg is implanted into the endometrium, falling levels of progesterone and oestrogen cause the lining to shed, leading to menses.

Panel 7.3: Suggested general reading and other resources

YouTube Channels

- Khan Academy: www.youtube.com/user/khanacademy
- Crash Course: Anatomy and Physiology: https://youtube/pVkUCrgQCCc?list=PL8dPuuaLjXtOAKed_MxxWBNaPno5h3Zs8
- Osmosis: www.youtube.com/@osmosis
- Armando Hasudungan: www.youtube.com/@armandohasudungan

Anatomy and Physiology textbook:
WAUGH, A. and A. GRANT, 2018. *Ross and Wilson anatomy and physiology in health and illness*. 13th ed. London: Elsevier.

Tips for studying anatomy and physiology

As mentioned at the beginning of this chapter, A&P is a vast subject and can be a daunting one for students with minimal experience in health science. This chapter briefly outlines the main systems of the human body; however, in your studies, you will most likely find that you are studying this topic in much greater detail.

Assessments in A&P modules can include both written assessments, including case studies and reports or include examinations that could include short answer or multiple-choice questions. Below are some tips for studying A&P more generally and some tips for writing A&P assignments.

- Break the subject down: as shown in this chapter, A&P can be split into different sections. These could be the six organisation levels of the human body or the different systems of the human body. By breaking the subject down, you can split a large subject into smaller more manageable chunks
- Repetition: repetition is one of the best tools when studying A&P. It may seem obvious, but the more often you look over a subject, the easier it becomes to remember, and understanding will follow. When studying A&P, repeatedly reading, writing and studying the material will help you
- Find what works for you: there is a wealth of resources available for you in A&P, ranging from academic textbooks, journals, YouTube videos and 3D programmes. Find what works for you and use it. Are you a visual learner who likes 3D models of the human body? Do you prefer reading and absorbing the material in academic textbooks? Do you prefer creating your own revision materials? Be honest about what works and does not work for you and use it to your advantage
- Be aware of your strengths and weaknesses: it is normal in A&P to prefer one system/ area over another. You may find the nervous system hard to understand but find the urinary system easy to understand. Concentrate on your weaknesses in your revision. If there is a certain area you struggle with, then spend your time focusing on this
- Use the correct terminology: you may find that there are certain words and phrases used in healthcare science that you are unfamiliar with. Part of being a practitioner is using this terminology, and it will be expected in your assignments. Make a glossary for this terminology and start using it in your practice and while studying
- Time: give yourself ample time for study and revision. This subject is not something that can be learnt overnight. Ensure that you give yourself time to complete the materials and set a schedule with a realistic time frame for you to incorporate study into your day

Summary

We explored A&P in this chapter, focusing on the organisation of the human body, the different human systems and key A&P concepts such as homeostasis and cell structure. Each of the different systems was examined in terms of its physiology and anatomy. The final section of the chapter provided tips for students studying A&P. Students are advised to break this subject down to understand it, be aware of their strengths and weaknesses and allow sufficient time to learn about the complex working system of the human body.

Box 7.5: Key learning points

- The human body can be split into six levels of structural organisation, moving from the smallest structure to the human body as a whole
- Cells are the smallest unit that make up all living things

- Homeostasis refers to the maintenance of internal bodily conditions in the face of constantly changing internal and external variables
- The nervous system is the body's primary command centre, and it collects information from both the internal and external environments, interprets this information and responds accordingly
- The function of the cardiovascular system is to maintain a continuous blood flow to all body cells to ensure an adequate supply of oxygen and other nutrients to maintain homeostasis and ensure optimum body functioning
- The circulatory system is made of a network of blood vessels comprising arteries and veins of varying sizes
- The digestive system's primary task is to convert dietary food into nutrients and energy, which our cells and body systems can use for all functions
- The musculoskeletal system consists of bones and soft tissues—tendons, ligaments, cartilage and muscles—which provide a framework for the body, allowing for movement, posture and body weight balance
- Break anatomy and physiology down to understand it. In this way, you can split a large subject into smaller and more manageable chunks.

Reference

WAUGH, A. and A. GRANT, 2018. *Ross and Wilson anatomy and physiology in health and illness*. 13th ed. London: Elsevier.

8 Caring for people with long-term conditions and multimorbidity

A health and social care perspective

Lindsay Welch

Box 8.1: Contents

- Introduction
- What are long-term conditions?
- A brief overview of the main long-term conditions and their clinical management
- Complexity through multimorbidity: The comorbidome
- Self-management of long-term conditions and the role of technology
- Long-term conditions in a broader context: Management and models of care

---

Box 8.2: Learning outcomes

By the end of this chapter, you should be able to

- Define long-term conditions
- Briefly explain the pathophysiology and clinical management of three common long-term conditions
- Identify the impact that long-term conditions have on individuals, their families, the wider society and health and social care
- Understand the importance of the biopsychosocial model in the care and management of people with long-term conditions
- Develop strategies to support people with long-term conditions and complex multimorbid pathologies.

DOI: 10.4324/9781003198338-11

Box 8.3: Keywords

- Long-term condition
- Self-care and self-management of long-term conditions
- Comorbidome
- Biopsychosocial model
- Digital technology

Introduction

This chapter will introduce the concept of long-term conditions (LTCs), explain why it is important to study these and to understand who is affected by LTCs. This chapter will support you to identify people with LTCs and to understand their conditions as well as their broader health and social care (H&SC) needs. Examples of common conditions and how these are treated or managed will be discussed and the wider societal and economic impact of LTCs will be explored. We will consider the role of an individual in their own care (this is called 'self-care' or 'self-management'), as this is an increasingly important, and debated, development in the treatment of LTCs.

What are long-term conditions?

LTCs are conditions that cannot be cured but can be controlled by medicines or other treatments and therapies (Department of Health 2012). The number of people in the population with one or more LTCs is growing. It is reported that approximately 19 million adults in the United Kingdom (UK) currently live with a LTC (ONS 2020), and one in four adults live with two or more LTCs (Budge, Taylor and Curtis 2021). These include physical health problems such as heart disease and lung disease, or physical and mental health problems such as depression and cardiac disease. Having one or more LTCs can have a significant effect on a person's ability to work and live a full life (Department of Health 2012). People are constrained by the long-term limitations caused by the symptoms of their own health conditions. These include poor mobility due to breathlessness or polypharmacy and complexities in medication regimes owing to having one or more LTCs (Czubak, Tucker and Zarowitz 2004).

The increase in LTCs has implications for the National Health Service (NHS) and access to usual care provision. People with LTCs account for 50% of all general practice appointments and 64% of all outpatient appointments. Seventy per cent of the total health care spend in England is attributed to caring for people with LTCs (Department of Health 2012).

Globally, the prevalence of LTCs is also rising, disproportionally in low-income countries (Hajat and Stein 2018). Moreover, there is an increase in people having one or more LTCs. These individuals are classed as having multiple LTCs or 'multimorbidity'.

Understanding LTCs and how to support people affected by them is a key area of H&SC practice. As H&SC professionals, it's important to be aware that many people have permanent, physically or psychologically life-limiting conditions, ones that requires adjustment to daily activities to stay as symptom-free as possible. Therefore, learning about LTCs – how they present clinically; how they can be treated and the impact they have on people, their families and the wider society – is a fundamental part of your learning in H&SC.

A brief overview of the main long-term conditions and their clinical management

---

Panel 8.1: Keywords and definitions

- Pathophysiology: abnormal physiology (Cambridge Dictionary 2022)
- Aetiology: the cause or causal factors of the disease (Cambridge Dictionary 2022)
- Symptoms/disease presentation: the subjective experiences of the person with the disease
- Treatment/management: Methods or mechanisms of lessening or reducing symptoms of the disease (Schrijvers 2009).

There are many LTCs, some occurring more frequently than others, so here, we will focus on the more common LTCs affecting each body system. These descriptions are by no means exhaustive; they are designed to provide an overview of some of the most common LTCs. Each condition will be described in terms of pathophysiology, aetiology, presentation and symptoms and treatment and management options.

Cardiovascular disease and coronary heart disease

Coronary heart disease (CHD) can also be referred to as 'ischaemic heart disease' or 'coronary artery disease'. Cardiovascular diseases (CVDs)—principally ischemic heart disease and stroke—are the leading cause of global mortality and a major contributor to disability (Roth *et al.* 2020). CVD is responsible for 10% of disability-adjusted life years (DALYs) lost in low- and middle-income countries and 18% of DALYs lost in high- to middle-income countries. The global CHD burden is projected to be at 82 million DALYs by 2020 (World Health Organization 2016).

Pathophysiology

CHD is characterised by a build-up of plaques (fatty materials) in the arteries. These plaques can form larger atheroma and can either stick to the side of vessel (artery) walls or break off and mix with other cells to obstruct the vessels entirely (blood clots).

Aetiology

The aetiology of this condition is multifactorial and is related to factors causing the build-up of fatty plaques as well as factors that increase the likelihood of plaques sticking to vessel walls. These include high cholesterol levels (more lipids [fats] circulating in the bloodstream), being overweight (higher levels of free fatty molecules) and high blood pressure (increased pressure can be from constricted vessels, as well and atherosclerosis). High blood pressure also increases the likelihood of clotting. Smoking increases blood coagulation, and the nicotine found in the cigarette also narrows down the blood vessels further, thus increasing the risk of clot formation.

CHD is also linked to family history (genetic links), age and ethnicity.

Symptoms/disease presentation

When the blood vessels become narrow in a person with CHD, this can initially cause symptoms of angina, such as tightening sensation or pain in the chest. The patient may also feel faint and experience breathlessness and nausea. Often, these symptoms are missed, and people know they have CHD only when they experience a full cardiac or vascular event, such as myocardial infarction or a cerebrovascular accident.

Treatment/management

Early identification of risk factors is important in CHD. This is through health screening, which can include checking for blood pressure and cholesterol. The modifiable risk factors must then be reduced; this might include intervening to promote weight loss, exercise and smoking cessation. This is the first part of CHD management and helps reduce the risk of a cardiac or vascular event.

However, once a patient has experienced a cardiac event, rapid and more invasive treatment is required. This can include surgery such as coronary angioplasty or bypass surgery (to bypass the clot).

Activity 8.1: Ticker Tapes

Listen to *Ticker Tapes* (https://www.bhf.org.uk/informationsupport/support/podca sts), the British Heart Foundation's podcasts that feature celebrities talking about their early diagnosis with heart disease and their personal experiences of heart surgery. These can be accessed at https://podcasts.apple.com/gb/podcast/celebrity-spec ial-graeme-souness-story/id1497174143?i=1000528297123.

Once the cardiac muscle dies (or becomes ischemic), that part of the heart loses its strength and function. In this case, long-term medications are required to support the weaker heart. These include medications to improve the strength and force of contractions or reduce the pressure of blood going into the heart.

The weaker heart does cause circulatory issues, particularly in the blood flow back to the heart, resulting in fluid pooling in the lower limbs. A careful mix of exercise and rest can support cardiac function and maintain circulation. Complex interventions for and education about LTC management are also necessary.

Chronic obstructive pulmonary disease

Chronic obstructive pulmonary disease (COPD) is the term used to describe long-term, obstructive (where a patient feels that they are unable to get the air out of their lungs) lung conditions.

COPD is the third leading cause of death in the world. Twelve per cent of the general population globally experience COPD (Varmaghani *et al.* 2019). The prevalence of COPD is increasing; a rate of 8.9% was reported in 2016 (Varmaghani *et al.* 2019). In 2015, COPD contributed to 2.6% of DALYs globally (GBD 2015 Chronic Respiratory Disease Collaborators 2017).

Pathophysiology

COPD is characterised by the destruction of parenchymal lung tissue. This can result is two pathophysiological processes, both of which overlap at times, and to different extents, in different people. Either the cells break down and become flattened (or 'baggy') and no longer have the potential to perform gas exchange, or there is an inflammatory response, causing excessive secretions and permanent airway constriction.

Aetiology

Smoking and ambient particulate matter are the main risk factors for COPD, followed by household air pollution, occupational particulates, ozone and exposure to second-hand smoke (GBD 2015 Chronic Respiratory Disease Collaborators 2017).

Symptoms/disease presentation

COPD typically presents as persistent breathlessness, which worsens on exertion, cough and sputum production (Global Initiative for Chronic Obstructive Lung Disease 2020).

Treatment/management

COPD is treated with a range of inhalation therapies, oral steroids and antibiotics during a flare up or exacerbation. Health behavioural changes (especially smoking cessation) are also recommended to slow down the progression of the disease. However, strength building and exercise are also part of the gold standard of care (Nici and Zuwallack 2014).

COPD is burdensome and disabling to live with because of the persistent breathlessness associated with it. Social support groups and charitable trusts can provide opportunities for people with COPD and their families to gain information and support.

Activity 8.2: Explore Breathe Easy support groups

Look at some of the group models of 'Breathe Easy' support groups across the United Kingdom. These can be seen at www.blf.org.uk/breathe-easy/Breathe-easy-models

Think about what people affected by chronic obstructive pulmonary disease gain from being a group environment as compared to managing their disease alone.

Diabetes mellitus

Diabetes mellitus (DM) is an endocrine or metabolic disorder. It can be categorised as type 1 or type 2 DM. Type 1 DM is characterised by the inability to produce or release insulin. Type 2 DM is more common and characterised by hyperglycaemia (high blood glucose), insulin resistance and insulin deficiency (Baynest 2015).

It is estimated that 415 million people around the world are living with DM, that is, nearly one in 11 people of the world's population. In the UK, it is estimated that around 3.5 million people have this condition, as some people remain undiagnosed (Diabetes.co.uk 2021). The prevalence of DM continues to increase, with an estimated 80% of people with DM living in low- to middle-income countries (Baynest 2015).

Pathophysiology

In type 1 DM, the pancreas stops making insulin because the cells preparing insulin (Islets of Langerhans) are destroyed by the body's immune system. If the body stops producing insulin, then glucose (sugar) cannot be transformed into energy to be used up by the body's cells, and it is left 'free floating' around the body (Galicia-Garcia et al. 2020).

Type 2 DM is one of the most common metabolic disorders and is caused by a combination of two factors: defective insulin secretion by pancreatic β-cells and the inability of insulin-sensitive tissues to respond appropriately to insulin (Galicia-Garcia et al. 2020).

DM is associated with complications such as CVD, nephropathy, retinopathy and neuropathy. It can lead to chronic comorbidities and mortality.

Aetiology

In the case of type 1 DM, a person is unable to produce sufficient insulin, so this is considered an 'idiopathic' LTC, and the person's own body causes this condition. Type 2 DM is often experienced later in life, as the body stops responding effectively to its own insulin and is no longer able to use blood glucose for regular function, thus causing blood glucose levels to become elevated (this is called 'hyperglycaemia') (Diabetes. co.uk 2021).

Symptoms/disease presentation

DM symptoms are related to high levels of circulating blood glucose and can include excessive thirst, frequent urination, sensation of hunger (even when eating), blurred vision, extreme fatigue, slow healing, weight loss (in type 1 DM) and tingling sensation, pain and numbness in the hands and feet (in type 2 DM).

Treatment/management

The treatment for DM depends on the level of support needed for the body to absorb insulin. Management approaches are designed to stabilise blood glucose at a low level (range: 5–7 millimoles per litre) to ensure the circulating glucose does not damage the cells, tissues and organs. If not managed well, DM can cause damage to large blood vessels, leading to atherosclerosis (commonly associated with hypertension), hyperlipid-aemia and obesity (Baynest 2015).

Treatment can involve the injection of insulin, modification of diet or medication to enhance the efficacy of insulin (Diabetes.co.uk 2021).

Activity 8.3: Carb counting

Explore the practice of 'carb counting' as part of the management of diabetes mellitus. Read this webpage: www.diabetes.co.uk/diet/carbohydrate-counting. html, designed to support people with diabetes, and watch the YouTube clip. Reflect on the adaptations, complications and benefits of this form of dietary management.

Complexity through multimorbidity: The comorbidome

Thus far, we have discussed common individual LTCs, their pathophysiology, aeti-ology, presentation and symptoms and treatment or management. It important to examine how to care and support someone who has more than one LTC. Multiple LTCs are burdensome for the affected people. Often, the symptoms of LTCs overlap, and it is difficult to ascertain the cause of symptoms such as pain, breathlessness and fatigue. This uncertainty can lead to feelings of being out of control and a sense of helplessness, which often feed further symptoms such as anxiety and low mood (or depression).

LTCs are often clustered around failing bodily systems, so, for example, CVDs can be connected to hypertension, with heart diseases likely being clustered. Studies of cardio-respiratory disease—COPD, in particular—have found that people with COPD have an increased prevalence of CVDs, psychiatric diseases and other comorbid conditions. This may be due to the causal lifestyle factors that contribute to the condition, such as smoking, ageing or genetic factors. In the case of COPD, comorbid conditions increase as the disease progresses.

This association of symptoms has been studied in people with COPD and has led to the development of the concept of the 'comorbidome', which is used to describe the rela-tionship between conditions, with each having an impact on the original condition, thus adding to the burden of symptoms and complexity of disease management. See Figure 8.1 for an illustration of the comorbidome for COPD.

In Figure 8.1, the area of each circle reflects the prevalence of the disease. The prox-imity to the centre (which represents mortality) expresses the strength of the association between the disease and risk of death (Almagro *et al.* 2012, 2015).

Therefore, the larger the bubble, the more likely you are, if you have COPD, to have the other condition. So, you would have a very high likelihood of acquiring cardiac issues such as arterial hypertension and atrial fibrillation. However, you are not very likely to have dementia and COPD but, if you do, then you would have the highest risk of mortality.

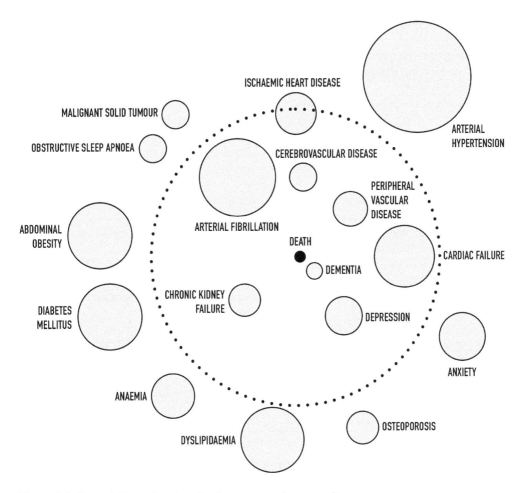

Figure 8.1 Comorbidome for chronic obstructive pulmonary disease
Image credit: Tamsin Arai Drake, adapted from: Almagro *et al.* (2012, 2015)

This concept can be applied to other LTCs such as neurogenerative diseases. A patient with a neurogenerative disease will likely have reduced physical movement and probably struggle to maintain an adequate nutritional intake. Given this, there is likely to be a 'knock-on' effect on bone density (which may, by itself, increase the risk of developing osteoporosis). This patient will experience an increase in disabling symptoms rather than early mortality (Visser *et al.* 2004).

Studies into multiple LTCs often focus on mortality outcomes and the contribution of other conditions to premature death. However, attention must also be paid to high levels of pain, mobility issues and overall poor quality of life experienced by people with multiple LTCs. Multi-disease also means multiple treatments, multiple appointments and interaction with multiple specialist health professionals.

Activity 8.4: How would you help this patient?

Let's consider the person with multiple long-term conditions by exploring the 'work' of treating patients through the lens of those with the condition and those who care for them.

First, access the Healthtalk.org site and listen to some of the personal stories of living with multiple long-term conditions. The site can be accessed here: https://healthtalk.org/multimorbidities/the-personal-impact-of-multiple-health-problems

Then, consider the practice implications of caring for these patients. Imagine a patient who:

- Is taking multiple medications for his or her disease. These medicines have side effects for which more drugs must be prescribed
- Is prescribed medicines from the hospital and needs to collect these from the pharmacy and must remember to order repeat medication
- Struggles with symptoms such as pain, fatigue or reduced mobility, making travel challenging
- Has anxiety, which makes him or her forgetful and renders the retention of new information challenging.

This hypothetical patient has been advised by his or her healthcare professional to work on 'self-management' of their conditions and given information to improve their management skills.

Would you change the advice given? If so, how? What would you say or advise? What might you do to help this patient?

Self-management of long-term conditions and the role of technology

Self-management of long-term conditions

The concept of self-management briefly referred to in the activity above represents the dominant theory (and practice) of care for people with multiple LTCs; this affects all decisions about care and treatment of the person affected by LTCs. This emphasis could potentially dilute other aspects of disease management, such as social support.

Self-management of LTCs focuses on successfully managing, or coping with, long-term health needs (Potter *et al.* 2018). 'Coping', as a term, broadens the idea of simply managing the physical symptoms and 'work' of a disease, as it encompasses the emotional and social aspects of living well with multiple conditions.

Studies suggest that, to reach the stage of 'coping', or successful living with a LTC, a person has to move through as a series of stages, these have been defined by Ambrosio and colleagues (Ambrosio *et al.* 2015) as:

- Acceptance
- Coping
- Self-management

- Integration
- Adjustment

Ambrosio and colleagues refer to this as a cyclical, dynamic process that generates changes in a person's thinking and their approach to living.

Activity 8.5: Engage with research and reflect

To explore the ideas discussed above, read Ambrosio *et al.*'s (2015) paper: 'Living with chronic illness in adults: a concept analysis', available at: https://doi.org/ 10.1111/jocn.12827 (this is not an open access journal and requires a subscription) and Potter *et al.*'s work (2018): 'The context of coping: a qualitative exploration of underlying inequalities that influence health services support for people living with long-term conditions' available at: https://doi.org/10.1111/1467-9566.12624 (open access).

While you are reading, reflect on the complexity of the disease on a person's quality of life and overall well-being. Consider how, in your role as a healthcare professional, you can build considerations of these into your communication with patients or care planning. When you are ill, what helps you to cope and manage the illness?

Digital technologies, wearables and future technologies

The third decade of the 21st-century has seen healthcare and care services move rapidly into the digital realm. Technology is now widely used to support LTC management, although this has not (to date) fully embedded in usual care pathways (NHSX 2021).

Since 2020–2021, and because of the need to move to online working because of the COVID-19 pandemic, there has been an increasing reliance on digital tools in the management of LTCs. This move can be experienced as empowering and providing people with LTCs the ability to monitor and manage their own symptoms and gaining a better understanding of their conditions through engagement with online videos and apps.

Wearables are simply wearable technology containing bio-sensors to track 'digital biomarkers'. These include movement tracking, heart rate sensing and sleeping time. Sensors use geo-location tags to understand and monitor distance. Wearables can also prompt people to move more and warn or trigger if people do not move enough, thus supporting the element of self-management, or self-care (Nguyen 2010).

Future technologies targeting people with LTCs are emerging to support the clinical management of diseases through peer support networks (Kennedy *et al.* 2016), behavioural change for healthy lifestyles (Bloom *et al.* 2020; Band *et al.* 2017) and physical diagnostics and biological monitoring (Soni *et al.* 2022). The FreeStyle™ Libre, used in the management of type 1 DM, is a technological breakthrough to enable continuous monitoring of glucose in peripheral fluid without the need to draw a blood sample.

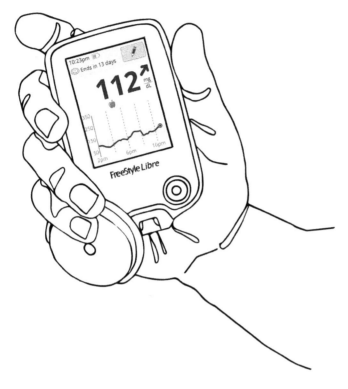

Figure 8.2 FreeStyle™ Libre
Image credit: Tamsin Arai Drake, adapted from: Soni *et al.* (2022)

Activity 8.6: Explore digital technology

Explore the use of digital technology for long-term condition management. Have a look on the App Store (www.apple.com/uk/app-store) on your iPhone to see what apps are available for the management of long-term conditions. If you have an Android phone, look at Google Play (https://play.google.com/store).

Long-term conditions in a broader context: management and models of care

LTCs, by their very nature, become part of every aspect of the lives of those affected. Healthcare professionals often consider only the physiological symptoms of illness and can sometimes forget about patients' social and psychological well-being.

One model that is particularly relevant for people managing LTCs (and for those caring them) is the biopsychosocial model (see Figure 8.4). This asserts that health and well-being are caused by a complex interaction of biological, psychological and sociocultural factors (Engel 1980).

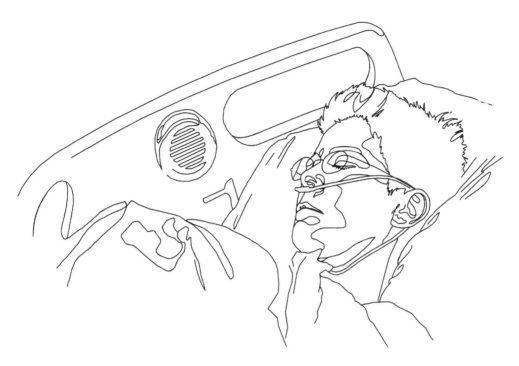

Figure 8.3 A patient being treated for a long-term condition
Image credit: Tamsin Arai Drake

The biopsychosocial model illustrates the interplay of the interactions of our moods, emotions, motivations, family support, community and society on our physical health. This relationship is multidimensional, as our physical health, particularly if you have an LTC, can impact your mental and social health and well-being (Engel 1979). People with LTCs often spend time negotiating health services and physically caring for themselves (taking medicines, ordering medicines, exercising, resting and eating well). All of these take time and energy. This time is increased in people with multiple LTCs and takes more effort in people who are fatigued or who are frail. Eliciting community support and working with local support groups can enable a sense of collective efficacy (Band *et al.* 2019). This sense of support when working together can support a person in managing their LTC, as well as fulfilling their social needs (bio-psycho-social).

Loneliness is a growing population issue. Communities of people are isolated, and communications are often online rather than face-to-face. This reduction in social activity, in turn, exacerbates mental health issues such as anxiety and depression (Cramm *et al.* 2012). Hopelessness, persistent symptoms, lack of mobility and low social interactions can lead to low mood and depression. Loneliness is a result of having LTCs, leading to issues with mobility, travel and expense, and it's also a precursor to the disease. Social isolation, loneliness and living alone have a significant and equivalent effect on the risk of mortality, which exceeds the risk associated with obesity (Holt-Lunstad 2017).

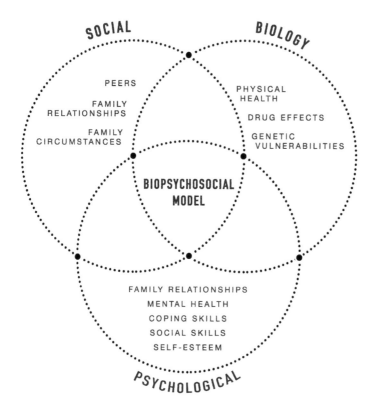

Figure 8.4 Biopsychosocial model
Image credit: Tamsin Arai Drake, adapted from: Engel (1979, 1980)

Therefore, community groups, linking people to support to manage their LTC, is vital for social, psychosocial and physical well-being.

NHS England has developed a model of care to advocate a broader paradigm (a considered perspective), based on the management of chronic conditions work undertaken by Wagner and Bodenheimer (Bodenheimer, Wagner and Grumbach 2002). The model has been referred to as the 'house of care' and devised to support primary care clinicians adapt key principles of care to their own area. It is based on six key principles:

1. People with LTCs are central to the process. They are supported by H&SC professionals to express their own needs and decide on their own priorities through a process of information-sharing, shared decision-making and action planning
2. Self-management support and the development of collaborative relationships between patients and professionals are at the heart of service delivery
3. Tackling health inequalities is a central aim of the house of care. The number of LTCs and their burden falls disproportionately on people with poor health literacy and those in lower socioeconomic groups. Tools, skills training and ongoing support must

be available to identify those who find it harder to engage with health issues and may need extra support to do so.

4. The house of care delivery system aims to ensure that each individual is involved in a unified, holistic care planning process with a single care plan. A common set of relevant skills and processes reduces the burden of training

5. Quality assurance of the philosophy, core approach and skills required is essential to ensure that implementation builds on relevant evidence and experiential knowledge, which is consistently applied

6. Care planning is the gateway to personalisation and/or personal health budgets

(Coulter, Roberts and Dixon 2013).

These key principles are being adapted and developed into local principles and practice to build a person-centred approach to LTC management.

Activity 8.7: Enabling people to live well for longer: 'What matters to you today?'

People's circumstances, beliefs and values matter in health and social care. They matter in understanding how we can make a true difference to people and improve their lives as they strive to cope with the management of long-term conditions. 'What matters to you? Is a Canadian initiative, a simple and effective way of communicating the fact that you intend to listen and act on patients' personal wishes and circumstances to improve control over physical and mental health conditions. Available at: https://bcpsqc.ca/advance-the-patient-voice/what-matters-to-you/

Activity 8.8: Clinical case study: Incontinence and breathlessness

Meet Valerie

Valerie is a 78-year-old lady. Valerie has a past medical history of:

- Severe chronic obstructive pulmonary disease (forced expiratory volume 30% of predicted)
- Osteoporosis
- Urinary incontinence
- Persistent lower back pain
- Wedge fractures of the spine

Valarie has reduced mobility and uses a mobility scooter. She is supported by her male cousin for transport and shopping but not for personal care. What do you think Valerie's main concerns and worries are? How could you support Valerie and help her manage her condition?

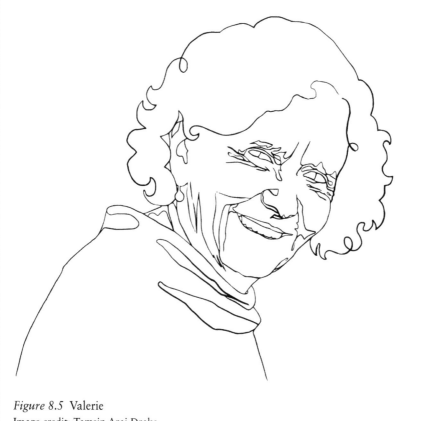

Figure 8.5 Valerie
Image credit: Tamsin Arai Drake

Activity 8.9: Reflect on the growth and prevalence of long-term conditions

Explore the differences and similarities in the aetiology and presentation of the long-term conditions discussed above. This King's Fund article is useful for this activity, which is available at: www.kingsfund.org.uk/projects/time-think-differen tly/trends-disease-and-disability-long-term-conditions-multi-morbidity

What features do all long-term conditions have in common? What are some of the main drivers of long-term conditions and why are they currently increasing in prevalence?

Summary

In summary, we have understood that living with LTCs is challenging and constraining, more so for people living with more than one condition. This chapter has explored multi-morbidity and the difficulties this poses to people in terms of personal care and self-management. There is a need to develop and implement person-centric models of care, coupled with emerging technologies, to empower people with LTCs to accept, cope and adapt to managing their multi-faceted health needs.

Box 8.4: Key learning points

- The prevalence of long-term conditions is increasing globally
- People often have more than one long-term condition. This means that their care and health need to be personally tailored to their needs and conditions
- Coronary heart disease is the leading global cause of mortality
- Chronic obstructive pulmonary disease is disabling and responsible for the loss of quality-adjusted life years globally
- The social and psychological needs of people with long-term conditions should be prioritised to enable people to successfully manage all aspects of their life and condition
- The biopsychosocial model illustrates the complex interplay between the differing aspects of long-term conditions
- Management of long-term conditions must prioritise the person to help them live well and to promote personal well-being.

References

ALMAGRO, P. *et al.*, 2012. Comorbidities and short-term prognosis in patients hospitalized for acute exacerbation of COPD: The EPOC en Servicios de medicina interna (ESMI) study. *Chest*, 142, 1126-1133. https://doi.org/10.1378/chest.11-2413

ALMAGRO, P. *et al.*, 2015. Comorbidome and short-term prognosis in hospitalised COPD patients: The ESMI study. *European respiratory journal*, 46, 850-853. https://doi.org/10.1183/09031936.00008015

AMBROSIO, L. *et al.*, 2015. Living with chronic illness in adults: A concept analysis. *Journal of clinical nursing*, 24, 2357-2367. https://doi.org/10.1111/jocn.12827

BAND, R. *et al.*, 2017. Intervention planning for a digital intervention for self-management of hypertension: A theory-, evidence- and person-based approach. *Implementation science*, 12, 25. https://doi.org/10.1186/s13012-017-0553-4

BAND, R. *et al.*, 2019. Development of a measure of collective efficacy within personal networks: A complement to self-efficacy in self-management support? *Patient education and counselling*, 102, 1389-1396. https://doi.org/10.1016/j.pec.2019.02.026

BAYNEST, H. W., 2015. Classification, pathophysiology, diagnosis and management of diabetes mellitus. *Journal of diabetes metabolism*, 6, 1-9. https://doi.org/10.4172/2155-6156.1000541

BLOOM, I. *et al.*, 2020. Findings from an exploration of a social network intervention to promote diet quality and health behaviours in older adults with COPD: A feasibility study. *Pilot and feasibility studies*, 6, 15. https://doi.org/10.1186/s40814-020-0553-z

BODENHEIMER, T., E. H. WAGNER and K. GRUMBACH, 2002. Improving primary care for patients with chronic illness: The chronic care model, part 2. *JAMA*, 288, 1909-1914. https://doi.org/10.1001/jama.288.15.1909

BUDGE, C., M. TAYLOR and C. CURTIS, 2021. Support for living well with long-term conditions: How people manage. *Journal of clinical nursing*, 30, 475-487. https://doi.org/10.1111/jocn.15560

COULTER, A., S. ROBERTS and A. DIXON, 2013. *Delivering better services for people with long-term conditions: Building the house of care*. London: The King's Fund.

CRAMM, J. M. *et al.*, 2021. The relationship between older adults' self-management abilities, well-being and depression. *European journal of ageing*, 9, 353-360. https://doi.org/10.1007/s10433-012-0237-5

CZUBAK, R., J. TUCKER and B. J. ZAROWITZ, 2004. Optimizing drug prescribing in managed care populations: Improving clinical and economic outcomes. *Disease management and health outcomes*, 12, 147-167. https://doi.org/10.2165/00115677-200412030-00002

DEPARTMENT OF HEALTH, 2012. *Long term conditions compendium of information*. 3rd edition. UK: Department of Health.

DIABETES.CO.UK, 2021. *Diabetes prevalence* [viewed 31 December 2022]. Available from: www.diabetes.co.uk/diabetes-prevalence.html

ENGEL, G. L., 1979. The biopsychosocial model and the education of health professionals. *General hospital psychiatry*, 1(2), 156-165. https://doi.org/10.1016/0163-8343(79)90062-8

ENGEL, G. L., 1980. The clinical application of the biopsychosocial model. *American journal psychiatry*, 137(5), 535-544. https://doi.org/10.1176/ajp.137.5.535

GALICIA-GARCIA, U. *et al.*, 2020. Pathophysiology of type 2 diabetes mellitus. *International journal of molecular sciences*, 21, 6275. https://doi.org/10.3390%2Fijms21176275

GBD 2015 Chronic Respiratory Disease Collaborators, 2017. Global, regional, and national deaths, prevalence, disability-adjusted life years, and years lived with disability for chronic obstructive pulmonary disease and asthma, 1990–2015: A systematic analysis for the Global Burden of Disease Study 2015. *The lancet respiratory medicine*, 5, 691-706. https://doi.org/10.1016/S2213-2600(17)30293-X

GLOBAL INITIATIVE FOR CHRONIC OBSTRUCTIVE LUNG DISEASE (GOLD), 2020. *Global strategy for the diagnosis, management, and prevention of chronic obstructive pulmonary disease (2021 report)*. WHO: Global Initiative for Chronic Obstructive Lung Disease.

HAJAT, C. and E. STEIN, 2018. The global burden of multiple chronic conditions: A narrative review. *Preventive medicine reports*, 12, 284-293. https://doi.org/10.1016/j.pmedr.2018.10.008

HOLT-LUNSTAD, J., 2017. The potential public health relevance of social isolation and loneliness: Prevalence, epidemiology, and risk factors. *Public policy and aging report*, 27, 127-130. https://doi.org/10.1093/ppar/prx030

KENNEDY, A. *et al.*, 2016. Implementing a social network intervention designed to enhance and diversify support for people with long-term conditions. A qualitative study. *Implementation science*, 11, 27. https://doi.org/10.1186/s13012-016-0384-8

NGUYEN, H. Q., 2010. Digital health consumers: Transforming the clinical research landscape. *Communicating nursing research*, 43, 29-43.

NHSX, 2021. NHSX delivery [Online] [viewed 31 December 2022]. Available from: www.nhsx.nhs.uk/about-us/nhsx-delivery/

NICI, L. and R. L. ZUWALLACK, 2014. Pulmonary rehabilitation: Definition, concept, and history. *Clinics in chest medicine*, 35, 279-282.

ONS, 2020. *People with long-term health conditions, UK: January to December 2019* [viewed 31 December 2022]. Available from: www.ons.gov.uk/peoplepopulationandcommunity/healthandsocialcare/conditionsanddiseases/adhocs/11478peoplewithlongtermhealthconditionsukjanuarytodecember2019

POTTER, C. M. *et al.*, 2018. The context of coping: A qualitative exploration of underlying inequalities that influence health services support for people living with long-term conditions. *Sociology of health and illness*, 40, 130-145 https://doi.org/10.1111/1467-9566.12624

ROTH, G. A. *et al.*, 2020. Global burden of cardiovascular diseases and risk factors, 1990–2019: Update from the GBD 2019 Study. *Journal of the American college of cardiology*, 76, 2982-3021. https://doi.org/10.1016/j.jacc.2020.11.010

SCHRIJVERS, G., 2009. Disease management: A proposal for a new definition. *International journal of integrated care*, 9, e06. https://doi.org/10.5334/ijic.301

SONI, A. *et al.*, 2022. A practical approach to continuous glucose monitoring (rtCGM) and FreeStyle Libre systems (isCGM) in children and young people with type 1 diabetes. *Diabetes research and clinical practice*, 184, 109196. https://doi.org/10.1016/j.diabres.2022.109196

VARMAGHANI, M., *et al.*, 2019. Global prevalence of chronic obstructive pulmonary disease: Systematic review and meta-analysis. *Eastern Mediterranean health journal*, 25(1), 47-57. https://doi.org/10.26719/emhj.18.014

VISSER, M. *et al.*, 2004. Assessing comorbidity in patients with Parkinson's disease. *Movement disorders*, 19, 824-828. https://doi.org/10.1002/mds.20060

WORLD HEALTH ORGANIZATION, 2016. *Global burden of coronary heart disease* [viewed 31 December 2022]. Available from: www.who.int/health-topics/cardiovascular-diseases.

9 Person-centred care

A paramount concept in health and social care

Teresa Corbett

Box 9.1: Contents

- Introduction
- What is person-centred care?
- A brief history of person-centred care
- Why does person-centred care matter in health and social care?
- Challenges in delivering person-centred care
- Using person-centred care in practice: Key concepts
- 21st-century person-centred care: Your role in promoting person-centred care

---

Box 9.2: Learning outcomes

By the end of this chapter, you should be able to

- Explore the concept of person-centred care
- Briefly describe the history of person-centred care in the United Kingdom
- Identify key concepts in person-centred care
- Consider its application in practice
- Critique current practice in person-centred care.

Box 9.3: Keywords

- Self-management support
- Shared decision-making
- Biopsychosocial model of health
- Values
- Self-actualisation
- Person-centred approach framework
- NHS Long-Term Plan

DOI: 10.4324/9781003198338-12

Introduction

When discussing the health and care of a person, we frequently refer to 'patients'. This is defined in the *Oxford English Dictionary* as: 'A person receiving or registered to receive medical treatment'. More and more people are now living with long-term conditions. Such conditions are often managed over many years outside of traditional centres of healthcare delivery and involve a variety of therapies and treatments. Thus, the lines between person and patient have become blurred over time. Given this, where does the *person* end and the *patient* begin?

Being a *patient* is just one of the many facets of an individual's life. Patients also include parents and grandparents, employees and caregivers, friends, lovers, neighbours, gardeners, choristers, football fans, musicians and many more. They have their own principles and standards, have experienced loves and losses and hold beliefs about what inspires them and keeps them motivated. This is true even of those who may not have the capacity to express such beliefs and may need advocates to voice their priorities on their behalf. If we focus on the individual solely as another patient, then we might forget these features of an individual. Focusing on this very narrow aspect of the person's life (that is, their role as a patient) devalues the individual's experience and, crucially, limits our ability to see the whole picture.

In this chapter, we will explore the concept of person-centred care (PCC) and consider its application in practice settings. The chapter will begin with a discussion of the history of PCC. Next, we will consider some of the challenges to implementing this type of care in practice and examine what types of key skills are required to deliver truly PCC. Finally, you will consider your role in promoting PCC as a practitioner.

Activity 9.1: Values and priorities

Before we explore the definitions of person-centred care, consider your core values and priorities. Think about 'what matters most to me?' Then make a list of your values and priorities. Consider how these values and priorities impact your day-to-day life and the decisions you have made. Have they influenced the choices you have made (for example, your career, your choice of partner, etc.)?

What is person-centred care?

The term 'person-centred care' has been used to describe several different ideologies and activities; however, there is no single agreed definition of the concept (Scholl *et al.* 2014). Below, we describe some of the key ideas underlying the philosophy of PCC.

PCC is a compassionate, holistic and empathetic approach to care delivery. Rather than healthcare delivered 'to' or 'for' people, PCC aims to promote healthcare 'with' individuals. Traditional one-size-fits-all models of care often neglect to include people in decisions about their care and primarily focus on clinical outcomes rather than the individual's priorities. PCC aims to deliver what many patient groups have often argued is necessary in care settings: 'what matters to someone' is not just 'what's the matter with someone' (NHS 2019a).

Panel 9.1: Core principles underpinning person-centred care

- Respect for an individual's values and priorities
- Supporting meaningful engagement
- Shared responsibility
- Ownership, autonomy and self-determination
- Understanding

Mezzich *et al.* (2010) summarise PCC as a philosophy that promotes care *of* the person, *for* the person, *by* the person and *with* the person. PCC is underpinned by values of mutual respect and understanding, as well as individual rights to self-determination (McCormack and McCance 2017, p.3). Emphasis is placed on the biography of the individual. The whole person is considered, including both negative and positive aspects of health and well-being; developing an understanding of a person's identity is central to how care is delivered.

PCC differs from many traditional approaches to healthcare delivery. It does not draw on a medical model of care. Instead, it promotes a multidisciplinary approach to care, acknowledging that individuals are likely to need a variety of professionals, as well as community groups and charities, to support them (Scholl *et al.* 2014). Such an approach challenges many of the traditional ways of working in health and social care (H&SC).

The philosophy of PCC promotes shared-control and shared-responsibility relating to decisions and management of health. The aim of PCC is to empower, enable and foster fulfilment in the person's life but doing so while working with clinicians. Individuals are equal, active partners in their care to ensure it meets their needs. They are not passive recipients of care delivery (Ham, Charles and Wellings 2018). Thus, the person is supported to develop the knowledge, skills and confidence to manage their own health and care.

Now that you understand what PCC is, let's look at how the concept has developed overtime.

A brief history of person-centred care

Coulter and Oldham (2016) began an exploration of the topic of PCC with the following quote from Hippocrates (a Greek physician known as 'The father of modern medicine'): 'It is more important to know what sort of person has a disease than to know what sort of disease a person has'. In this quote, Hippocrates touches on a point that is central to the concept of PCC: We need to know about the *person* who has the disease, not just what disease they have. In some ways, it seems like quite a modern view, but this was not always the prevailing view in H&SC. It might be that we have come full circle in how we think about health.

As noted previously, PCC places a focus on the patient as a whole person, addressing individual preferences and idiosyncratic needs while considering the social context in which a person lives. This is in contrast with traditional biomedical focus on a body part or disease. Traditional biomedical models of health and illness focus on the medical or biological causes of illness. As such, the medical professional was responsible for diagnosing and treating the condition, given their expertise and understanding of the pathogens involved in the disease. The individual was seen as a passive actor in the process of health and illness, and little consideration was given to ethical issues relating to autonomy, responsibility and dignity (McCormack *et al.* 2017). Traditional biomedical models are dominated by reductionism, a focus on disease, specialism and commercialism (McCormack *et al.* 2017).

However, with changes in our understanding, care professionals began to realise how other factors (apart from purely medical factors) could affect health. PCC is deeply linked to concepts proposed in humanistic psychotherapy (Hudon *et al.* 2011) and the work of Rogers (1952). Rogers used the term 'person-centred therapy', focusing more on the whole person rather than viewing a person as either a patient or a client. In *person*-centred therapy, relationships are based on a therapist's authenticity and capacity to empathise with the service user and to do in a non-judgemental way. The aim of such approaches is to help service users to work towards self-actualisation (this is about realising one's potential), building confidence and self-esteem while developing purposeful relationships with others (McCormack *et al.* 2017; Rogers 1959).

In the1960s, Virginia Henderson defined the function of a nurse as being to: assist the individual, sick or well, in the performance of those activities contributing to health or its recovery (or to peaceful death) that he would perform unaided if he had the necessary strength, will or knowledge. And to do this in such a way as to help him gain independence as rapidly as possible (Henderson 1964, p.63).

Henderson's definition captures key elements of PCC, including the focus on enabling and supporting the individual to work towards achieving their health-related goals (and Henderson's quote evokes the concept of self-actualisation promoted by Rogers).

By the 1970s, many individuals had started to reconsider the clinician-patient relationship and how health services impact patient empowerment. A prominent example of this shift in thinking was the creation of the biopsychosocial model of health promoted by George Engel (1977) (see Figure 8.4, chapter 8). The model incorporates the different factors that might play a role in the development and maintenance of illness (namely, biological, psychological and social factors). In a biopsychosocial model of health, the individual's role in the development of conditions is recognised (that is, the individual may be responsible for illness), but they also play a key role in the treatment and management of their conditions. Responsibility for treatment is not restricted only to the medical professional but is also shared with the service user, who is an active actor rather than a passive actor in managing their health.

Towards the end of the 20th century, thanks to medical and technological advances, individuals with chronic conditions began to live longer. Such conditions do not require acute care in a hospital setting. Individuals now often manage (multiple) physical and mental health conditions in the community for many years. The modern health system is challenged to address this, not only in terms of diagnosis and treatment but also in relation to prevention, rehabilitation and long-term care. Owing to limited healthcare resources, optimal utilisation of resources is key to ensure efficient and effective provision of care. The person (or patient) at the heart of the system is one such resource.

Since the early 2000s, healthcare systems have been encouraged to opt for more viable approaches to care, where individuals are engaged in healthcare and take responsibility for the maintenance of their well-being (for example, Wanless Report 2002). Health has been re-imagined as something that is co-created by the individual, the community and the healthcare system (Wagner 1998; Wallace 2012). In turn, the role of the H&SC professional has evolved to include ongoing support for self-management and the promotion of the maintenance of health outside of traditional medical settings. Such changes in our conceptualisation of health have ushered in a new era of patient involvement and the development of initiatives that seek to promote informed and shared decision-making.

In the next section, we will explore the impact of this evolution in healthcare delivery and explore why PCC matters in modern H&SC.

Why does person-centred care matter in health and social care?

Care for the individual has always been at the very heart of what H&SC work involves. However, PCC seeks to go beyond *providing* care, carefully embedding considerations of how contextual and personal factors influence the way in which care is delivered and received. At a global level, groups such as the World Health Organization place person- and people-centredness at the heart of their agenda, proposing that individuals, families and communities should be supported to participate in healthcare services that respond to their needs in holistic ways (World Health Organization 2015). Person-centred approaches such as self-management support and shared-decision making are increasingly embedded as part of routine clinical practice. Professional bodies increasingly recognise person-centred practices as a core competency. Why is this?

Western societies are increasingly individualised in every domain of life including healthcare (McCormack *et al.* 2017). Technological advances have enabled us to learn about the human genome; this has facilitated individualised treatment plans (so-called 'personalised or precision medicine'). By understanding people's genetic make-up and combining and analysing this information with other clinical and diagnostic information, patterns that can help identify and treat complex diseases can be determined. An example of this can be seen in modern cancer care where personalised therapy or immunotherapy drugs are being developed to target an individual's specific gene changes or proteins in cancer cells (Heinemann *et al.* 2013). Such drugs stop the growth and spread of some cancers by blocking the cancer-causing proteins or genes in cancer cells (NHS 2022).

However, while healthcare has become increasingly specialised and individualised in some ways due to novel treatment approaches such as whole-genome sequencing and greater use of patient data and informatics, it has not always succeeded in being *person-centred*, with the values and priorities of the patient at the core. Evidence suggests that allowing individuals to express thoughts, ideas and strategies that are important to them is central to optimising care (Sharma, Bamford and Dodman 2015). Healthcare professionals who can incorporate patient priorities and preferences can promote patient involvement in decision-making and promote patient self-determination.

When delivered appropriately, PCC can be extremely beneficial (Sharma, Bamford and Dodman 2015). Some of the potential multidimensional positive effects include improved outcomes and satisfaction for those receiving care and increased job satisfaction in those who provide care (Brownie and Nancarrow 2013). PCC can also improve continuity of care and increase collaboration across teams and healthcare settings.

Challenges in delivering person-centred care

Health services—including their organisational processes and systems—can present challenges to providing PCC. Crucially, the organisational culture of many H&SC settings can have a huge influence on whether clinicians feel supported, motivated and capable of working in a person-centred way. Disjointed information and technology systems and fragmented care can make it difficult to communicate information effectively with service users and their carers. More and more specialised healthcare systems mean that care is often siloed; people may need to see a variety of different healthcare professionals. This takes time and effort. Often, individuals must organise appointments and administration relating to their condition, yet poor communication or coordination across teams can exacerbate workload. An increased treatment burden can lead to poor adherence, wasted resources and poor outcomes.

Delivering PCC can be especially challenging in some contexts, such as settings where individuals with intellectual disabilities or cognitive impairment are cared for. These individuals can experience problems expressing themselves due to impairment or disability. However, evidence indicates that staff training on communication and a clear understanding of behaviours can enhance the experience of these individuals. In some cases, family members and caregivers might be involved in this process if assistance is sought by the person or if the person is unable to make decisions on their own (Downs 2013).

In the community, people are expected to take more responsibility for their own health. However, with this increased responsibility some have asked whether there is too much burden placed on the patient. People with long-term conditions must learn to manage complex treatment regimens and work to embed these regimens in their daily lives (May, Montori and Mair 2009). Consequently, there is an ongoing movement to reinstate the person at the centre of their healthcare, emphasising empowerment and the appropriate provision of support and information. May, Montori and Mair (2009) have called for minimally disruptive medicine and treatment regimens tailored to the realities of patients' daily lives. They suggest that coordination of care should be prioritised from the individual's perspective, as these individuals know how their health and healthcare management impacts their daily lives. As such, many advocates, scholars and practitioners have proposed that these people should be involved in making decisions about their care.

Activity 9.2: Case study: Person-centred care in practice

Read Ali's story and consider how person-centred care is demonstrated in her case.

Ali was recently diagnosed with multiple sclerosis. The news of this diagnosis was daunting. Ali did not know how she would cope if she could no longer go for a run to clear her head. She imagined her body seizing up and being confined to a wheelchair, isolating her from her friends and family. Over time, she developed a low mood and found daily tasks difficult.

Ali's general practitioner referred her to a structured education programme to help with her understanding the condition and the things that could be done to improve her self-management of the condition. Following a conversation with a staff member at the education programme, Ali realised it was helpful to talk about her feelings. She explained how she had lost motivation and told her running friends that she wasn't going to be able to run with them anymore. Ali was advised to access a local peer support group of people who shared similar experiences. She found this helpful and met people who had continued to run despite their diagnosis. Some people had taken up running after their diagnosis. Ali learned that everyone seemed to have different experiences of multiple sclerosis and that running might even help with some of the symptoms. She called up her friends and arranged to go running with them again.

As time progressed, Ali started reading more online about what she could do to delay symptom progression. She brought some notes with her to an appointment with her multiple sclerosis specialist nurse. Together with her nurse, Ali set a goal to try to stay active and independent for as long as possible. They broke this overarching goal into small steps and decided to prioritise her running, as it was an important coping strategy for her. The nurse also told Ali about the different ways in which running could potentially help her symptoms.

However, owing to her low mood and fluctuating symptoms, Ali found it increasingly difficult to go out for a run. The nurse suggested that Ali might benefit from meeting with a health coach to help her with her motivation and assist her to make small changes to help her stay active. They talked about how she would likely have good days and bad days and how she could learn to manage her emotions on days when running was not possible for her.

Ali was referred to a physiotherapist to ensure that she was stretching correctly before each of her runs to maintain flexibility and ease pain. Ali found this session motivating and encouraging, as the physiotherapist explained that even a gentle jog on a 'bad day' could help multiple sclerosis symptoms. Ali began to understand that she would need to get to know her symptoms and listen to her body.

However, one day she found that her symptoms had suddenly became worse, with feelings of numbness developing in her hands and face. She was very worried, so she contacted her multiple sclerosis specialist nurse. Ali was referred to a rehabilitation team who reassured her that such flare-ups were quite common. She discussed the different medications that could help her to manage the feelings of weakness and poor balance she was experiencing. Ali did not like the idea of taking a course of intravenous medications, so her nurse suggested that oral corticosteroids might work better for her.

After a short course of medication, Ali felt much better physically but was angry that she had so little control over her symptoms. She discussed the experience with her rehabilitation team and said she'd like to learn more about strategies to prevent future relapses. She found the education and information helpful. Ali learned about reputable charities and resources where she could find out more about multiple sclerosis. She started doing yoga to complement her running, and through this, she developed an interest in meditation. This helped her to feel like she was regaining control of her body and mind. Ali continued to run, training regularly with her friends. Her rehabilitation team was also able to put her in contact with a group of runners with multiple sclerosis. She found this group particularly motivating and encouraging and learned a lot from the experiences of those who had lived for many years with multiple sclerosis. Some had even gone on to race in marathons— Ali couldn't believe it! For the first time since her diagnosis, she felt that it could be a very long time before she would need a wheelchair and that she could still achieve a great deal.

Over the next few months, Ali developed the skills and confidence to self-manage her multiple sclerosis, gradually going for longer runs and managing her mood.

Using person-centred care in practice: Key concepts

PCC Approaches are founded on developing, coordinating and providing healthcare services that are centred on individuals' beliefs, values, desires and wishes. It is respectful and responsive, recognising the unique needs of an individual regardless of age, gender, faith, social status, ethnicity and cultural background. Practitioners must work with the person to plan and deliver care that takes account of their context (including their social context, community networks and material resources). A person-centred practitioner must also be flexible and adaptive, as the patient's priorities may change over time as their needs change. This is in contrast with many evidence-based practices that approach care-delivery in a context-free manner, removing considerations of the person's biography from the intervention being delivered. PCC is a collaborative, genuine partnership between the practitioner and the individual.

However, as noted above, it is not always easy to implement in practice. With limited time and space, it can be difficult for H&SC professionals to find the opportunity to engage in meaningful person-centred conversations with service users. In this section, we will look at how PCC can be used in everyday practice.

Panel 9.2: The comprehensive model for personalised care

This has six evidence-based and inter-linked components, each of which is defined by a standard, replicable delivery model. These include:

1. Shared decision-making
2. Personalised care and support planning
3. Enabling choice, including legal rights to choose
4. Social prescribing and community-based support
5. Supported self-management
6. Personal health budgets and integrated personal budgets

Adapted from: NHS (2019b).

Chapter 1 of the NHS Long-Term Plan (2019a) emphasises that personalised care should be standard practice across the health and care system. To achieve this, the Comprehensive Model for Personalised Care (NHS 2019b) was developed as a delivery plan for PCC (see Panel 9.2). The document was co-produced with people with lived experience and a wide range of stakeholders.

The person-centred approach framework (Fagan *et al.* 2017) aims to facilitate the delivery of Comprehensive Model for Personalised Care (see Figure 9.1).

It provides a core skills education and training framework to support practitioners. The framework was commissioned by Health Education England and outlines best practice and sets out key, transferable behaviours, knowledge and skills. These core skills aim to support people to feel connected, involved, empowered and supported. Values and communication and relationship-building skills are at the heart of this framework.

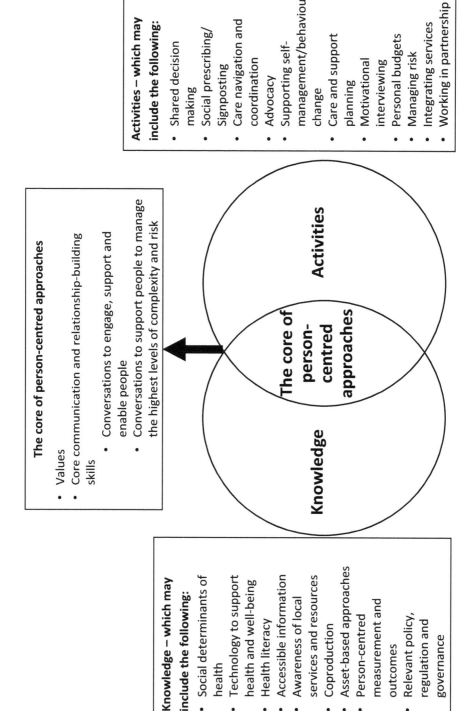

Activities – which may include the following:

- Shared decision making
- Social prescribing/Signposting
- Care navigation and coordination
- Advocacy
- Supporting self-management/behaviour change
- Care and support planning
- Motivational interviewing
- Personal budgets
- Managing risk
- Integrating services
- Working in partnership

The core of person-centred approaches

- Values
- Core communication and relationship-building skills
  - Conversations to engage, support and enable people
  - Conversations to support people to manage the highest levels of complexity and risk

Activities

The core of person-centred approaches

Knowledge

Knowledge – which may include the following:

- Social determinants of health
- Technology to support health and well-being
- Health literacy
- Accessible information
- Awareness of local services and resources
- Coproduction
- Asset-based approaches
- Person-centred measurement and outcomes
- Relevant policy, regulation and governance

Figure 9.1 Knowledge and activities of person-centred approaches
Adapted from: Fagan *et al.* (2017)
Image credit: Teresa Corbett

Values are the principles underpinning our attitudes. They are demonstrated in our behaviours (that is, what we say and do). Therefore, to deliver PCC, it is important to consider our own values and the values of the team we work in. We need to consider what matters to us and reflect on how these values impact our actions.

Activity 9.3: What matters to you?

Consider three values that are central to your practice
Why do these values matter?
Do work in line with your values? Think of examples of when your values have guided your work.

Examples of values that apply to people working in H&SC might include the following:

- I value treating people with respect, dignity and empathy, without judging them
- It is important to me to understand other people's preferences, viewpoints and priorities
- It is important to me to foster a rapport with the people I work with and to develop mutual trust in my interactions
- I appreciate the experiences of people and value their expertise
- I value co-production and working with people to improve the quality of services.

Core communication and relationship-building skills

Meaningful communication is central to the development of relationships between people. Within H&SC practice, meaningful communication enables us to help service users to feel respected and valued. By feeling listened to and having their perspective valued, people are more likely to feel supported and empowered.

Savundranayagam and Hummert (2004) label the consequences of inappropriate or poor communication as 'missed opportunities' to enhance care. As an illustration of how communication can lead to missed opportunities, consider the impact of healthcare professionals' use of directive language (for example, 'sit up', 'lie down', 'take off your shirt'). Such language can be perceived as giving orders or making demands and does not allow input from the person being treated (Connabeer 2021). These actions do not always facilitate a person-centred approach. Instead, a conversation is required that

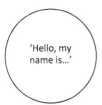

Figure 9.2 Hello my name is...
Image credit: Teresa Corbett

enables the clinician to understand what the individual wants, experiences, perceives, feels or understands.

Let's look at some things that you can do to improve your communication and relationship-building skills in practice.

Introduction

Dr Kate Granger was a doctor and a terminally ill patient with cancer. During a stay in the hospital, she noticed that many of those looking after her did not introduce themselves before delivering care.

This frustrated Kate and, in response, she started the 'Hello, my name is...' campaign through social media to remind the H&SC staff about the importance of introducing themselves. Kate argued that meaningful communication makes a huge difference to people, and this starts with a simple introduction (Granger 2013). By introducing yourself to the person you are caring for, you are treating them with respect. She campaigned with her husband to encourage H&SC staff to introduce themselves to those they are caring for.

You can incorporate this into your practice by providing your name, purpose and role at the beginning of interactions with service users. It is also helpful to give the other person the opportunity to introduce themselves. That way, you can find out simple things like what they like to be called.

The setting

Having meaningful conversations is central to providing PCC. However, we need to consider where and when to have those conversations.

For example, you might need to consider distractions such noise or lighting, which may reduce the person's ability to see or hear you. You should also consider privacy; people may not feel comfortable sharing their experiences if they think they will be overheard. A familiar and comfortable location is more likely to put someone at ease. If you are arranging to meet someone, then it is important to make sure that there are no accessibility issues that may pose a barrier to them. Consider the positioning of chairs and tables in the room. If you are too close to them, they might feel that you are invading their personal space. Chairs that are too low or uncomfortable can pose difficulties for individuals, but you should also ensure that the chairs are turned to face each other to minimise twisting and turning.

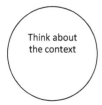

Figure 9.3 Think about the context
Image credit: Teresa Corbett

In your next interaction with a service user, consider the setting and whether it is the appropriate place for a conversation.

Communication

When we think about communication, we often initially think about *verbal* communication. This relates to what we say, and it influences the rapport we develop with someone. Also, *what* you say and *how you say it* are also important.

In a person-centred approach to care, it is helpful to adopt an empathetic and compassionate style of communication. At the start of a consultation, it can be helpful to clarify the purpose, aims and priorities of the encounter. As with introductions, this helps to manage expectations and facilitate a sense of co-production and active partnership between the clinician and the patient or service user. To foster this, check whether there is anything else the person would like to discuss during the consultation. It can also be useful to ask before you offer advice, to check that the person knows already and what they would like to know. This shows respect for the individual and acknowledges that they may have some pre-existing expertise and their own opinions about managing their health. It can be helpful to adopt an open style of questioning to encourage the individual to speak about their experiences. This can be achieved by posing questions that do not have a simple 'yes' or 'no' answer. You might also want to acknowledge any emotions you are perceiving in the patient or mention what you notice about the way the person describes their experience. This serves as a form of reflection and indicates to the individual that you have heard them and understood what they have said.

While what we say is important, most interpersonal communication is expressed through largely unconscious nonverbal behaviours (an estimated 60%–65% according to Burgoon, Floyd and Guerrero (2010)).

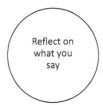

Figure 9.4 Reflect on what you say
Image credit: Teresa Corbett

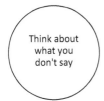

Figure 9.5 Think about what you don't say
Image credit: Teresa Corbett

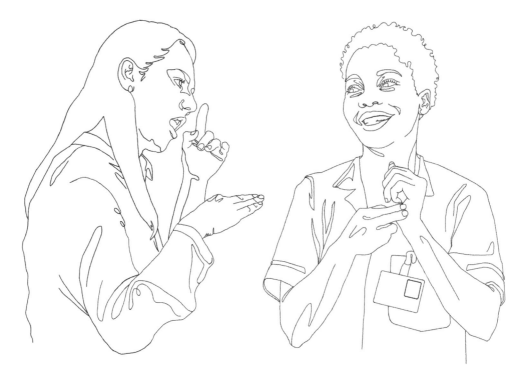

Figure 9.6 Nonverbal communication
Image credit: Tamsin Arai Drake

We use our body to provide a signal to others, conveying a thought, emotion or awareness through physical gestures, posture and facial expressions. However, one of the most powerful nonverbal cues is the use of silence. In a person-centred interaction, this can allow an individual to process their thoughts, think of what they want to say and allow them the time to say it. As well as facilitating reflection, a practitioner's silence might also signal to the other person that they should lead the interaction or explain a point in more detail. Silence can create the space for people to express their feelings. Maintaining silence can convey empathy. For example, a person might become quiet because they are feeling emotional. By maintaining the silence, the practitioner is indicating that they recognise the emotions of the other person and are giving them the time to process their feelings.

By becoming aware of your own nonverbal cues, you can enhance your practice. Attending to how you communicate nonverbally can help you to identify ways to improve rapport with service users. In your practice, it can be useful to reflect on how you communicate different types of information to different people; in what way does your approach change, depending on the context?

Active listening

One of the most important elements of a truly person-centred interaction is to consider *how* you listen.

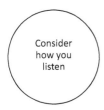

Figure 9.7 Consider how you listen
Image credit: Teresa Corbett

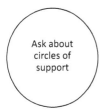

Figure 9.8 Ask about circles of support
Image credit: Teresa Corbett

It is one of the most effective ways to understand another person's perspective and is a skill you can continue to develop over the course of your career. To be an active listener, you must lay your assumptions to one side and demonstrate a completely focused willingness to engage with the person who is speaking. This helps to indicate a genuine interest in what they have to say. Active listening takes a lot of concentration and requires the practitioner to be fully present, attending socially, emotionally and psychologically to what is being said. Successful active listening not only demonstrates your interest but also helps to gain trust. Crucially, as a practitioner, it will also enable you to gather information to facilitate a deeper understanding of what the person is talking about. Ensuring that you hear and understand will help you to promote involvement and facilitate open discussion and reflection.

Finding out who else is supporting the individual

In describing conversations between H&SC professionals, service users and carers, it is important to recognise the many connections and resources people may draw upon.

Individuals, friends, family and communities have their own unique expertise and strengths to offer. Drawing 'circles of support' can help us consider the value and importance of a variety of community assets and resources supporting us, or those of an individual we are trying to support. The important thing to consider is not the number of people in the social network but the quality of those relationships.

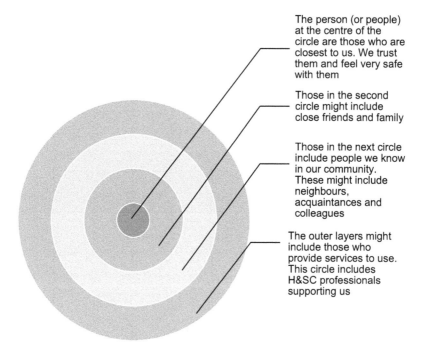

The person (or people) at the centre of the circle are those who are closest to us. We trust them and feel very safe with them

Those in the second circle might include close friends and family

Those in the next circle include people we know in our community. These might include neighbours, acquaintances and colleagues

The outer layers might include those who provide services to use. This circle includes H&SC professionals supporting us

Figure 9.9 Circle of closeness
Image credit: Teresa Corbett, adapted from: Fagan *et al.* (2017)

Activity 9.4: Circles of support

Draw your circles of support. Map the people who are present in your life and with whom you interact with on a regular basis. Consider how close they are to you. After completing this task, you will have an overview of the relationships that have the greatest influence on your life, and who you can ask for support for different kinds of issues. Consider why it might be useful for H&SC professionals to find out this information about service users and patients.

21st-century person-centred care: Your role in promoting person-centred care

Moving forward, a one-size-fits-all health and care system will struggle to meet the increasing complexity demanded of healthcare. The NHS Long-Term Plan (2019a) was published to outline the strategic plan for the National Health Service (NHS) over the next 10 years. The Long-Term Plan identifies five practical changes to the NHS model, one of which emphasises the importance of delivering person-centred and personalised care: 'People will get more control over their own health, and more personalised care when they need it' (p.24).

Professional standards of practice and behaviour for nurses, midwives and nursing associates (Nursing and Midwifery Council 2018) require registered practitioners to prioritise the interests of service users. This encompasses ensuring that their dignity is maintained, and needs are recognised, assessed and responded to. People receiving care should be treated with respect and listened to. The guidelines emphasise that registered nursing practitioners avoid: 'Making assumptions and recognise diversity and individual choice' (Nursing and Midwifery Council code 1.3, Nursing and Midwifery Council 2018). Further, practitioners should respond to peoples' preferences and concerns, working in partnership with them to ensure effective care delivery. As such, the contribution that people can make to their own health and well-being is recognised and respected. People should be encouraged and empowered to share in decisions about their treatment and care. When joining the Nursing and Midwifery Council register, nurses, midwives and nursing associates commit to upholding these standards which are a fundamental elemental part of the profession.

Activity 9.5: '... people will never forget how you made them feel'

Maya Angelou has written: 'People will forget what you said, people will forget what you did, but people will never forget how you made them feel'.
    Reflect on how this quote relates to person-centred approaches to care delivery?

As Miles and Asbridge (2019) note, PCC is 'here to stay'. It is not an abstract concept, ethical debate or a moral standpoint. Instead, it signals a radical shift in practice that is strongly justified based on a wealth of scientific evidence and ethical and economic principles. Yet, translation into practice has been a criticism of the ambitious aims of the NHS Long-Term Plan. There are still several barriers to developing and embedding PCC as part of routine healthcare. There is no quick fix, especially within a complex system like the NHS.

As mentioned previously, PCC does not ignore traditional medical models but incorporates psychological and social approaches to develop healthcare practice for the 21st-century. As a new generation of graduates entering the workforce, you will be required to bring a 'new way of thinking and doing' to your role, challenge the *status quo* and draw on a novel set of skills to support this novel approach to care. Even as you begin your career, you can encourage and empower fellow colleagues to be more person-centred in their approaches. As outlined earlier in the chapter, strategies such as 'Hello my name is...' and the practice of active listening can have a great impact on the rapport with a service user and do not take much time to implement.

Self-awareness and participation in reflective practice key in PCC. As you develop your skillset, it will be important to incorporate ongoing reflection in your practice. You will need to think about your own experiences, knowledge and feedback you receive from others (including supervisors, colleagues and patients). It will also be important to continually evaluate how your own values and beliefs are incorporated into your clinical practice. When you reflect, you should consider the extent to which you have respected patients and service users' roles in their care and incorporated their views, skills, resources and experiences into it. In placements, it might be helpful to keep a diary or discuss your person-centred approach with colleagues. It would also be helpful to seek mentorship and feedback about this aspect of your practice.

The ambition in the Long-Term Plan is for PCC to support as many people as possible. As this movement of person-centred approaches and personalised care evolves in the future, you will have a key role to play in its success.

Summary

In this chapter, you have learned about what PCC means and how the concept has developed over time. We have also explored some of the challenges associated with the implementation and delivery of PCC. By exploring key concepts and skills, you have been encouraged to reflect on your own practice and think deeply about how you can integrate person-centred approaches into your role. Looking to the future of care, we have considered the aims of professional bodies and organisations such as the NHS, who promote the importance of placing the individual at the heart of their care.

Box 9.4: Key learning points

- Person-centred care aims to promote the autonomy of the individual and ensure that 'what matters' to them is a central consideration in their care. The philosophy of person-centred care promotes shared-control and shared-responsibility relating to decision and management of health
- Person-centred care presents a shift in thinking from traditional biomedical models of healthcare that were often reductionist and disease-focused. The person-centred care approach goes beyond providing care; it also considers how contextual and personal factors influence the way in which care is delivered and received
- Allowing individuals to express their thoughts, ideas and strategies that are important to them is central to optimising care
- Delivering person-centred care can be challenging owing to siloed and disjointed healthcare services. It can be difficult also to ensure ongoing consideration of the preferences of those who have trouble expressing themselves due to impairment or disability
- Despite these challenges, research indicates that there are wide-ranging benefits of providing person-centred care, including improved outcomes and satisfaction for those receiving care and greater job satisfaction among those providing care
- Person-centred care is founded on developing, coordinating and providing healthcare services centred on individuals' beliefs, values, desires and wishes. It is respectful and responsive, as well as flexible and adaptive
- Key skills in person-centred care include communication and relationship-building skills, as well as the ability to engage in a variety of activities including shared decision-making, personalised care and support planning and supported self-management
- The NHS Long-Term Plan emphasises the importance of delivering person-centred care as one of the five practical changes to the NHS model. It aims person-centred care to support as many people as possible
- Self-awareness and participation in reflective practice are central in person-centred care

References

BROWNIE, S. and S. NANCARROW, 2013. Effects of person-centered care on residents and staff in aged-care facilities: A systematic review. *Clinical interventions in aging*, 8, 1-10. https://doi.org/10.2147/CIA.S38589

BURGOON, J. K., K. FLOYD and L. K. GUERRERO, 2010. Nonverbal communication theories of interpersonal adaptation. In: C.R. Berger, M.E. Roloff and D.R., Roskos-Ewoldsen, eds. *The handbook of communication science*. 3rd ed. Thousand Oaks, CA: Sage Publications, pp.93-110.

CONNABEER, K., 2021. Lifestyle advice in UK primary care consultations: Doctors' use of conditional forms of advice. *Patient education and counseling*, 104(11), 2706-2715. https://doi.org/10.1016/j.pec.2021.03.033

COULTER, A. and J. OLDHAM, 2016. Person-centred care: what is it and how do we get there? *Future hospital journal*, 3(2), 114. https://doi.org/10.7861/futurehosp.3-2-114

DOWNS, M., 2013. Putting people-and compassion-first: The United Kingdom's approach to person-centered care for individuals with dementia. *Generations*, 37(3), 53-59.

ENGEL, G. L., 1977. The need for a new medical model: A challenge for biomedicine. *Science*, 196(4286), 129-136. https://doi.org/10.1126/science.847460

FAGAN, P. et al., 2017. *Person-centred approaches: Empowering people in their lives and communities to enable an upgrade in prevention, wellbeing, health, care and support*. London: Health Education England, Skills for Health and Skills for Care [viewed 30 May 2022]. Available from: www.skillsforhealth.org.uk/wp-content/uploads/2021/01/Person-Centred-Approaches-Framework.pdf

GRANGER, K., 2013. Healthcare staff must properly introduce themselves to patients. *BMJ*, 347:f5833. https://doi.org/10.1136/bmj.f5833

HAM, C., A. CHARLES and D. WELLINGS, 2018. *Shared responsibility for health: The cultural change we need*. The King's Fund [viewed 30 May 2022]. Available from: www.kingsfund.org.uk/publications/shared-responsibility-health

HEINEMANN, V. et al., 2013. Targeted therapy in metastatic colorectal cancer–An example of personalised medicine in action. *Cancer treatment reviews*, 39(6), 592-601. https://doi.org/10.1016/j.ctrv.2012.12.011

HENDERSON, V., 1964. The nature of nursing. *The American journal of nursing*, 64(8), 62-68.

HUDON, C. et al., 2011. Measuring patients' perceptions of patient-centered care: A systematic review of tools for family medicine. *The annals of family medicine*, 9(2), 155-164. https://doi.org/10.1370/afm.1226

MAY, C., V. M. MONTORI and F. S. MAIR, 2009. We need minimally disruptive medicine. *BMJ*, 339, b2803. https://doi.org/10.1136/bmj.b2803

MCCORMACK, B. and T. MCCANCE, 2017. Chapter 1 - introduction. In: B. McCormack and T. McCance, eds. *Person-centred practice in nursing and health care: Theory and practice*. Chichester, UK: John Wiley and Sons, 1-9.

MCCORMACK, B. et al., 2017. Person-centredness in healthcare policy, practice and research. *Person-centred healthcare research*, 3-17. https://doi.org/10.1002/9781119099635.ch1

MEZZICH, J. E. et al., 2010. Conceptual explorations on person-centered medicine 2010: Introduction to conceptual explorations on person-centered medicine. *International journal of integrated care*, 10, e002. https://doi.org/10.5334%2Fijic.472

MILES, A. and J. E. ASBRIDGE, 2019. The NHS long term plan (2019): Is it person-centered? *European journal for person centered healthcare*, 7(1), 1-11.

NHS, 2022. *Personalised medicine* [viewed 21 April 2022]. Available from: www.england.nhs.uk/healthcare-science/personalisedmedicine

NHS, 2019a. *The NHS long term plan* [viewed 21 April 2022]. Available from: www.longtermplan.nhs.uk/online-version/chapter-1-a-new-service-model-for-the-21st-century/

NHS, 2019b. *Comprehensive model for personalised care* [viewed 21 April 2022]. Available from: www.england.nhs.uk/publication/comprehensive-model-of-personalised-care/

NURSING AND MIDWIFERY COUNCIL, 2018. *The code: Professional standards of practice and behaviour for nurses, midwives and nursing associates* [viewed 25 September 2022]. Available from: www.nmc.org.uk/standards/code/

ROGERS, C. R., 1952. 'Client-centered' psychotherapy. *Scientific American*, 187(5), 66-75.

ROGERS, C. R., 1959. A theory of therapy and personality change. *A theory of therapy, personality, and interpersonal relationships: As developed in the client-centered framework.* New York: McGraw-Hill. Vol. 3, pp.212-220.

SAVUNDRANAYAGAM, M. Y. and M. L. HUMMERT, 2004. Creating caregiver identity: The role of communication problems associated with dementia. *Language matters: communication, identity, and culture*, 325-353. https://10.1177/0164027509351473

SCHOLL, I. *et al.*, 2014. An integrative model of patient-centeredness–a systematic review and concept analysis. *PloS one*, 9(9), e107828. https://doi.org/10.1371/journal.pone.0107828

SHARMA, T., M. BAMFORD and D. DODMAN, 2015. Person-centred care: An overview of reviews. *Contemporary nurse*, 51(2-3), 107-120. https://doi.org/10.1080/10376 178.2016.1150192

WAGNER, E. H., 1998. Chronic disease management: What will it take to improve care for chronic illness? *Effective clinical practice*, 1(1), 2-4.

WALLACE, L., 2012. *Co-creating health: Evaluation of the first phase*. London: The Health Foundation [viewed 30 May 2022]. Available from: www.health.org.uk/sites/default/files/CoCreatingHealthEvaluationOfFirstPhase.pdf

WANLESS, D., 2002. *Securing our future health: Taking a long-term view*. London: HM Treasury [viewed 21 April 2022]. Available from: citeseerx.ist.psu.edu/viewdoc/download?doi=10.1.1.471.8987&rep=rep1&type=pdf

WORLD HEALTH ORGANIZATION, 2015. *WHO global strategy on people-centred and integrated health services: Interim report*. Geneva: World Health Organization [viewed 21 April 2022]. Available from: apps.who.int/iris/bitstream/handle/10665/155002/WHO_HIS_SDS_2015.6_eng.pdf?sequence=1&isAllowed=y

10 Service user involvement in education

Kieron Hatton and Margaret Johanson

Box 10.1: Contents

- Introduction
- The development of service user involvement in the United Kingdom
- Service user involvement in social work education
- Conceptualising the involvement of people using services
- Creating new forms of power and meaningful change
- Service user involvement and social pedagogy
- Service user experiences

Box 10.2: Learning outcomes

By the end of this chapter, you should be able to

- Understand the concept of 'service user'
- Appreciate the way service user involvement arose out of the struggles of people who felt disempowered by their treatment by welfare professionals
- Understand how power operates and the impact of power differentials on service users
- Engage with the voices of people with real-world experience of working with welfare professionals.

Box 10.3 Keywords

- Service users
- Carers
- Creativity
- Power
- Social pedagogy
- Lived experience of service users

DOI: 10.4324/9781003198338-13

Introduction

From somewhat limited beginnings, service user involvement has become central to the accreditation and validation of social work and allied health professionals practice programmes (Hatton 2015). However, the extent and depth of service user involvement varies widely across the country and in many, but not all, cases focuses on the involvement of service users in the more traditional elements of such programmes including participating in admissions interviews, guest teaching and acting as an expert speaker.

This chapter argues that, if we are to make service involvement meaningful, we need to develop a more holistic and complex way of understanding how service users can contribute to social work and health and social care (H&SC) education. To achieve this, this chapter argues that we need a more developed analysis of power, imagination and creativity.

Why is understanding service user perspectives important for social work and H&SC students? For two main reasons. First, students will encounter service users while on their programmes of study. As noted above, service users are often involved in admissions processes, and many students may have been interviewed by a service user while applying to their programme of study. Many students are also likely to have heard service users speak about their experiences on a professional development day. Second, H&SC and social work students will be caring for service users and their carers once qualified (or, as in the case of apprentices, while they are studying). It's therefore imperative that they understand the unique perspective of service users.

A note on terminology

The term 'service user' is used here, although we fully recognise that (a) service users are not a homogeneous grouping and (b) that the very term itself is contentious (McLaughlin 2009). In current discussions, service users (as well as their carers) are more often referred to as 'experts by experience' or 'people with lived experience'. The authors also recognise that service users have multiple identities beyond their status as service users and that many of these roles intersect (Hill Collins and Bilge 2016) and cause contradictions or conflicts. This is the content of a companion piece (see Hatton 2020).

The development of service user involvement in the United Kingdom

Over the last 20 years, service users have at last been recognised as having a significant role in the delivery, management and development of welfare services. This is reflected in the attention given to service user involvement in both legislative and policy contexts. These debates cut across all service boundaries and raise questions about service user representation (Hatton 2015), the efficacy of current initiatives and the usefulness of the service user perspective across a range of service user areas.

The drivers behind these initiatives have often been service users themselves. The role of disability activists in creating the political climate to support anti-discriminatory legislation around disability is well known (Shakespeare 2013), as was their role in ensuring that the *Disability Discrimination Act 1995* (subsequently the *Equality Act 2010*) was amended to give disabled people the right to enforcement action if their entitlements were not met.

Recently, the development of services incorporating personalisation (see Social Care Institute for Excellence 2011) and co-production (see Social Care Institute for Excellence 2022) has proved an important motor for this enhanced move towards empowering people in the adult social care sector. Such an approach was further developed in the proposals around co-production, which has placed the emphasis on users and user-led organisations. The Social Care Institute for Excellence (SCIE) has produced a guide to co-production, which suggests that it is possible to identify some key features that are present. Co-production, they suggest, define(s) people who use services as assets with skills and break(s) down the barriers between people who use services and professionals.

Three features of personalisation—design, commission and delivery—are critical to our ability to distinguish whether service user involvement has any meaning or not. Equally, the key elements of co-production involve promoting people's strengths, reciprocity and mutuality, and the idea of people as change agents. Ideas of co-production, in particular, link closely to the concerns within this chapter about how we develop 'meaningful' ways of securing the involvement of service user in the delivery of social work and H&SC education.

Service user involvement in social work education

Within social work, there has been a clear articulation of the importance of securing service user involvement (Anghel and Ramon 2009). This is reflected in teaching (Waterson and Morris 2005), assessment and peer review (Humphreys 2005; Skoura-Kirk *et al.* 2013), face-to-face interactions between service users and students and the use of video and other tools (Waterson and Morris 2005). As Irvine, Molyneux and Gillman (2015, p.148) argue, the students they looked at had a strong perception that their practice was improved by input from service users and carers (see also reflections below).

Activity 10.1: How is service user involvement promoted in your workplace?

How is service user involvement promoted and supported in one of the organisations within which you have worked? Was this meaningful or did you feel that the organisation paid only lip service to the idea. Was it real or tokenistic? (see also: Arnstein 1969).

The Portsmouth experience

The Social Work Inclusion Group (SWIG) at the University of Portsmouth has been established in slightly different forms since June 2004 with support of money provided by the General Social Care Council (and latterly the Department of Health) with the aim of securing the involvement of service users in the design and delivery of programmes. At Portsmouth, this involvement has taken a variety of forms including:

- Interviewing and admissions procedures
- Teaching—the group was one of the pilot groups chosen by *Skills for Care* to deliver a training programme to train service users to teach on the Portsmouth social work degree programme

- Redesigning the curricula
- Assessing students 'readiness for practice' at the end of the first year of undergraduate study or first semester of postgraduate study
- Producing a video ('What I want from a social worker') and a series of DVDs
- Assessing student presentations
- Developing a range of drama and cultural activities for use in social work training
- Assessing presentations by applicants seeking academic positions
- Small-scale research around homelessness—Working with ex-street homeless people and homelessness organisations as co-researcher
- Auditing work placements
- Designing an audit tool to assess whether placement agencies meet students' learning needs
- Attending and contributing to team meetings
- Attending and contributing to course validation and other events

(Hatton 2017).

Service user involvement in the social work programmes in Portsmouth has as its central aim the development of creative teaching artefacts to engage with students in a critical and empowering way. These will be considered now.

Creative teaching materials

The example of the *CREATE* day (part of the BSc programme) demonstrates how the aim of producing a creative artefact was achieved through the co-production of activities by students, service users and staff.

Inspiration for the potential outcomes was often initiated by service users, with the students then coming on board to work out how to best achieve the suggested outcomes, using film, theatre, dance, poetry or other forms of performance. The staff offered facilitative support to achieve the desired outcomes which was delivered by students and service users in small group presentations to the whole cohort.

The BSc students were also asked to engage in a debate day in which two groups presented different aspects of a key issue facing service users. The groups were co-facilitated by a member of SWIG and a member of the academic staff. The students were allocated to groups, so they would sometimes be asked to present arguments that they may not have been supportive of. Such an approach encouraged students to step out of their comfort zone, research and engage with ideas they may not have been familiar with. The combination of these activities developed the students' critical abilities and their confidence in engaging and communicating with service users in a way the presence of service users as teachers (an approach also used) could not replicate.

The *Perspectives Project* sought to adopt a similar approach. Students, service users and carers, in a small group, co-produced a piece of theatre, film or similar artefact that was presented to the whole year group on a presentation day. The outcomes were often powerful and gave a 'voice' to service users/carers who are often under-represented in academic discourses (for example, see: swig.uk.net).

Activity 10.2: Creativity

What do you understand by creativity? How can you use creativity in your practice? Would a more creative approach to practice enhance the services you work in? If so, how?

Conceptualising the involvement of people using services

The theoretical underpinning for involving people using services in social work and H&SC education has frequently been under-conceptualised. Generally, involvement has been seen as good and part of a broader inclusion agenda that seeks to engage with the empowerment of people using services. It has focused on the importance of power relationships (Tew 2006), and the need for service user 'voice' (Beresford 2013) and has been critical of managerialist and procedural approaches to engagement with people using social work services particularly in the age of austerity (Jordan and Drakeford 2012).

However, these areas could be further developed. Power discourses have drawn on a range of writers from across the social and political sciences. Foucault (1991) reminds us that power operates in a complex way and that we need to deepen our understanding of power at macro and micro levels. He argues that:

> [T]he problems which I try to address ... which involve daily life, cannot be easily resolved. It takes many years, decades of work carried out at grass roots level with the people directly involved, and *the right to speech and political imagination must be returned to them* ... the complexity of the problem will be able to appear in its connection with people's lives ... the object is to proceed a little at a time, to introduce modifications that are capable of, if not finding a solution, then at least changing the givens of a problem (p.158-159, emphasis added).

While Foucault was addressing issues of political power in the broad sense, his comments can just as easily be seen as a prime legitimation for our concern with involving people who use services. Work with service users and carers is specifically about releasing people's *political imagination* so that they can envision an alternative experience, a different way of experiencing and delivering welfare and social work services. It is also about focusing on the particular daily experience of those people most directly involved in delivering social work services. It is concerned with changing the way issues are framed so that service users are not seen as 'problems' or 'clients' but rather as active partners in changing the services they directly experience.

Engaging and creating partnerships with people who use services has a change dimension; it is essentially political, which means that when examining service user involvement, we need to ask if the involvement we are discussing is real or tokenistic (Webber and Robinson 2012). To achieve real inclusion and engagement, we need to have a multi-dimensional concept of power, which incorporates a range of factors as illustrated in Figure 10.1.

This conceptualisation of power includes inclusion and participation, the link between theory and practice, the achievement of personal and political power through creativity and artistic action and an underpinning commitment to the recognition of agency (people's ability to act for themselves) as the determining factor in people realising their

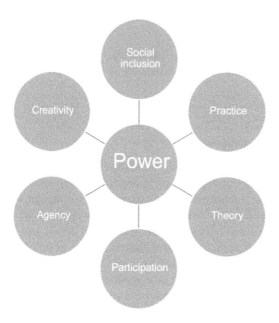

Figure 10.1 Dynamic view of power
Adapted from: Hatton (2017)

potential. This involves the recognition that service users are not victims who receive negative treatment by services, but people who have the ability and capacity to make changes themselves and to be active participants in that process.

SWIG members attribute great importance to their having a significant role in training and educating social workers. Their concern is not just to highlight issues but to contribute to the development and improvement of services. Such an involvement is essential if services are to be able to meet the demands placed on them in the evolving welfare state.

Creating new forms of power and meaningful change

Gramsci (1971) maintained that the ruling classes dominate through a mixture of force and consent, where the consent is gained through assuming the political, moral and intellectual leadership in the society. Such groups maintain control by making their rule and the legitimacy of state rule appear 'common sense'. It is then the role of external agents such as intellectuals, union organisers and community leaders (and in the context of this chapter—service users) to challenge this common sense.

Without an analysis of the way in which ideas are transmitted, we reproduce an analysis that suggests that service users are passive in the face of the power of large social work or professional welfare agencies. From this reading of Gramsci, we can see that service users struggling to have their voices heard are themselves acting as agents of change.

How can we acknowledge the capacity of service users to take action to gain power rather than have power handed to them? We can do this by seeing service users as people with the capacity to bring about change not only in their own, individual circumstances, but within the broader institutions and structures against which they struggle. Empowerment, therefore, becomes central to the service user experience (Hatton 2015).

To make involvement and participation real, we need to look not just at how power can be exercised but also at how it can be resisted. How can we develop strategies to promote meaningful change? Giddens refers to power as 'the transformative capacity of human action' (Cassell 1993, p.109). This is the key element in the notion of 'praxis'. Praxis is the creation of a radical practice, based on ideas of overcoming oppression, tackling discrimination and oppression and the creation of new cooperative social relationships that are at the heart of any theory of social action. Similar ideas can also be seen in Freire's idea of 'conscientisation', the notion that when the person becomes aware of the way their oppression is determined, they develop the capacity to take action to change their situation (Freire 1972; Gramsci 1971).

Power should be viewed as a dynamic concept in which individuals 'are always in the position of simultaneously undergoing and exercising ... power [they] are the vehicles of power, not its application' (Foucault 1980, p.98). This is the agency that we, as social workers, allied health professionals, academicians and service users, are looking for. This is the idea that service users can resist and reframe their experience in a way that makes a meaningful change to the way services are delivered. However, it is necessary to avoid an outcome in which the primary benefits are to the organisation rather than to the service user.

There is a need to identify why people act or fail to act to redress any disadvantage they experience. Underpinning the need for a focus on participation and inclusion is a commitment to recognise the agency of service users.

Fook (2002, p.200) has characterised this as a 'sense of responsibility, of agency, an appreciation of how each player can act upon it to influence a situation'. Central to this is the development of a consciousness, which can imagine another different way of doing things, a point similar to that attributed to Foucault earlier in this chapter (Foucault 1980). Hatton (2015) has suggested that this would enable, 'the creation of a radical practice based on notions of overcoming oppression... and the creation of new co-operative social relationships, (which are) at the heart of any theory of social action' (p.113).

Activity 10.3: Understanding power

What do you understand by power? Why is this important when we are working with service users? How can we support service users to become empowered?

Service user involvement and social pedagogy

One way in which this can be seen is through the prism of the European concept of social pedagogy (Hatton 2013), which is defined by Hamalainen (2003) as, 'to promote people's social functioning, inclusion, participation, social identity and social competence as members of society' (p.76). This commitment to social action is recognised as a central tenet of social pedagogy by several writers (Hatton 2013). This is also reflected in Vygotsky's idea of the 'creative imagination', which occurs 'whenever a person imagines, combines, alters and creates something new' (Vygotsky 2004, p.11). This will involve setting agendas for change, not just responding to the agenda of those with power (Jordan and Drakeford 2012).

Central to a pedagogue's activity is the use of *head, heart and hands*. The *head* enables the pedagogue to develop an understanding of the reasons for their intervention, the *heart* indicates the regard for and empathy with the person or group with whom the pedagogue is intervening and the *hands* indicate the range of practical activity and creativity that the pedagogue uses in any intervention (Boddy and Statham 2009).

It is now widely accepted that a focus on inclusion is central to good social professional practice (Beresford and Hoban 2005; Hatton 2015, 2017). Those involved in radical social and community work will appreciate the difficulty of achieving real inclusion rather than the often-tokenistic attempts at inclusion that agencies seek to perpetuate (Arnstein 1969; Ferguson and Woodward 2009; Hatton 2015).

Activity 10.4: What do you understand by social pedagogy?

What do you understand by social pedagogy? Why is this important when we are working with service users/carers? Consider the relevance of the idea of '*head, hands* and *heart*' to your current and/or future professional practice?

It is now recognised by the institutions of the state (Government departments and the new regulator of social work—*Social Work England*), higher education institutions, academics, students and users of welfare services that the involvement of service users in social work and H&SC education is a good thing. To continue to develop an understanding of this, it's important to recognise the dynamics of power relationships, the need for inclusion and the centrality of the service user 'voice'.

We will now consider how these more theoretical reflections relate to the lived experience of people using services.

Service user experiences

Margaret

As co-author of this article, Margaret has reflected on the way her experience illustrates some of the themes discussed above. Margaret reflects that, to experience a true sense of involvement in the education and training of social workers and H&SC professionals, the service user needs to be not an adjunct to, but a part of the team. She says:

> I think that the service user should be included as part of the team. The aim of any social or healthcare professional is to care for the person and their thoughts, and even ideas should be taken into consideration.

This, she suggests, means service users becoming equal partners in the development of approaches to resolve the issues she and other service users face when accessing care.

Thinking of the educational experience, Margaret observes:

As a person who suffers from fibromyalgia and most of its symptoms, I think it's important to have someone like me involved in the student's journey. I can provide a first-hand account of how debilitating a long-term condition can be, especially one that isn't visible or commonplace. Talking to the students, explaining symptoms, medication, medical bias, society's perception amongst other things can make the difference when they are in their workplace, and they come across someone with a similar health condition.

Margaret provides a powerful example of how useful this approach is:

For example, a few years ago, I was asked to come in and do a talk on chronic pain. Once I had explained my pain and the medication I take, the students told me that they had a better understanding of how pain, day in and day out, can not only change the patient's life but also the lives of all those around them.

The inclusion of service user perspectives, Margaret suggests, should begin at the point of recruitment:

At interview stage, you get a feel for those prospective students who are naturally empathetic and/or caring who feel the right fit for a career in health care. I always think 'would I be happy for this person to be taking care of me?'

Margaret's 'back story' informs her attitude to the inclusion of service user perspectives on H&SC and social work programmes. She says that:

It took many years for me to get a diagnosis, as my doctor repeatedly told me I was imagining everything, which was very demoralising and, in fact, made my symptoms worse. After seeing a locum doctor for something unrelated, they noticed that I'd been struggling with back pain, fatigue and insomnia. They said that they were concerned there might be some underlying health condition that wasn't showing up on blood tests or X-rays, so they referred me to a rheumatologist. Within a few months, I had been diagnosed with fibromyalgia, referred to a pain clinic and put on a medicine regimen. If it hadn't been for the locum looking at my medical history as a whole, rather than just being a lot of random problems, I probably wouldn't even be able to work today. It only took one doctor to have a proper conversation with me to make me feel valued and that I wasn't just wasting everyone's time.

Margaret argues that, for welfare professionals:

Communication is the most powerful tool anyone can have—both positive and negative. The need to be able to communicate with everyone (not just the people you like) is key. Communication isn't just about talking, it's about engaging with people, sometimes even a 'good morning' said with a smile is enough to make someone's day.

The reframing of service users' experiences in ways that recognise services users' ability to identify the issues they face is reflected in her hospital experience:

We all know that you can't get on with everyone, but all that anyone wants is to be treated with respect and dignity, and communication is at the centre of this. Whilst in hospital, there was a lady two beds down from me. For three nights, she screamed and shouted, and the staff (and patients) just kept telling her to go to sleep. This one night, this lady was very loud again. One of the nurses came in and asked if she'd like to go and have a cup of tea and a chat, as there was obviously something making her so distressed. They went off together only for about 10 minutes, the lady came back calm and went to bed. After that, there was no further screaming or shouting from her in the night and became a model patient. All it took was one short conversation and she was happy.

As Margaret notes:

No one wants to be in a hospital, a care home, the doctors or any other medical situation; however, it's a sad fact of life that, at one time or another, all of us will need some, if not all, of these services. Each environment differs; however, they all have one thing in common—(we are all) human beings. It may not always be easy to explain to a service user, especially if they are distressed or confused, but taking a few extra minutes just to try to provide some reassurance can make all the difference.

Margaret draws on these experiences in her interactions with students:

Talking to the students and being able to provide my own patient-centred view from my experiences, I think is very important so that they can see the way communication has an impact on the patient, both positively and negatively. All of us are service users at one time or another, and it is important to remember to treat each other with respect whether you are the service user or healthcare professional.

Despite some of the problems Margaret has encountered in the past, she remains optimistic about the progress being made when she states that:

I think that these days healthcare professionals are more willing to engage and are no longer shrouded in mystery or as aloof as they were in the past, so, generally, people feel more in control of their own care, and this can provide a more positive outlook to recovery or acceptance of a diagnosis.

However, she cautions:

It is important to remember that not every interaction with service users will go to plan. There is no 'one-size-fits-all' approach to communication. Some people like the bare facts given to them, while others want to know exactly what everything means down to the last detail, and some others are somewhere in between. Know your audience and adapt your approach accordingly.

In relation to working with students, Margaret's final observation is a resoundingly positive one:

On a personal note, I have found that sharing my experiences with our wonderful students has helped my mental health. I have found myself discussing things that

I didn't know and had been bottling up and some things that I had totally forgot. The only conclusion I can make is that the students made a safe space for me so that I was able to speak without fear of judgement or repercussions, and whilst it is always an exhausting exercise, it is also invaluable both for the student and for myself.

Activity 10.5: Think of a time when you or a member of your family or friends have had contact with a health or social care professional

Think of a time when you or a member of your family or friends have had contact with a health or social care professional.

- How did they make you/them feel?
- Was it a good or bad experience?
- If you had been the healthcare or social care professional, is there anything you would have done differently?
- Is there anything you can take from the experience to improve/help how you interact with service users in the future?

Service users and staff at the University of Portsmouth

Margaret's reflections are echoed in accounts of service users and staff at the University of Portsmouth. Their reflections on their own experience of creatively interacting with each other point to several ways in which service user involvement in educational programmes can enhance learning experience. Service users observed that:

The reason we do creative work is that it has proved to be the best way to educate future social workers...it isn't until they sit down and see life through our eyes that they get a real understanding of the issues around social work.

If you want to change the way social work operates...it is time to start listening to (us). It's not until they put themselves in our place that they realise the impact of bad practice and accept that they wouldn't put up with it.

When asked, social work students reflected that:

Co-producing creative artefacts led (us) to see (service users) differently. And seeing people with a disability not as people with disabilities but just as people...it's more than just tokenistic. It's actually from the get-go, working together, coming up with ideas together. Producing what you produce together. And really using the service user's knowledge, their skills, to come up with something at the end.

Another student noted that:

Service users are heard, but, for some reason, their 'voice' gets lost further down the process...this creative work has (taught me) that, as social workers, we need to be challenging managers and higher authorities and say, 'well OK, but the service users say this'.

Summary

This chapter explored service user involvement in social work and H&SC programmes. We argued that we need to develop a more holistic and complex way of understanding how service users can contribute to social work and H&SC education in ways that are not tokenistic. We drew on our experiences of being a social work academic engaged in activities to promote service user involvement at one UK university as well as the lived experiences of one service user with a chronic condition, Margaret. What Margaret and Portsmouth University service users and students share is a belief that service user involvement in education is a confirmation of the ability of service users to draw on their own understandings and capacity to promote and (hopefully) achieve real change for themselves. That they can, in a nutshell, demonstrate capacity. In addition, the work undertaken in Portsmouth (and other universities) demonstrates that people's creativity and imagination can be utilised to provide new, unique sand insightful educational experiences, which can, we believe, transform the way care will be delivered in the future.

Box 10.4: Key learning points

- Service user involvement presents an opportunity to hear the 'voice' of service users and to understand how they experience services
- Service user involvement is central to accreditation and validation of social work and allied health professionals practice programmes
- Involving service users is seen as part of a broader inclusion agenda, which seeks to engage with the empowerment of people using services
- Understanding power is a key factor in service user involvement
- There is a need to develop a more holistic and complex way of understanding how service users can contribute to social work and health and social work education in ways that are not tokenistic.

References

ANGHEL, R. and S. RAMON, 2009. Service users and carers' involvement in social work education: Lessons from an English case study. *European journal of social work*, 12, 185-199. https://doi.org/10.1080/13691450802567416

ARNSTEIN, S., 1969. A ladder of citizen participation. *Journal of the American institute of planners*, 35(4), 214-224. https://doi.org/10.1080/01944366908977225

BERESFORD, P., 2013. Service user issues: Rights, needs and responsibilities, in B. Littlechild and R. Smith, eds. *A handbook for inter-professional practice in the human services: Learning to work together*. Harlow: Pearson, pp.187-199.

BERESFORD, P. and M. HOBAM, 2005. *Participation in anti-poverty and regeneration work and research: Overcoming barriers and creating opportunities*. York: Joseph Rowntree Foundation.

BODDY, J. and J. STATHAM, 2009. *European perspectives on social work: Models of education and professional roles*. London: Thomas Coram Research Unit, Institute of Education.

CASSELL, P., ed., 1993. *The Giddens reader*. Basingstoke: Macmillan.

FERGUSON, I. and R. WOODWARD, 2009. *Radical social work in practice: Making a difference*. Bristol: Policy Press.

FOOK, J., 2002. *Social work: Critical theory and practice*. London: Sage Publishers.

FOUCAULT, M., 1980. *Power/knowledge: Selected interviews and other writings*. Brighton: Harvester Wheatsheaf.

FOUCAULT, M., 1991. *Remarks on Marx*. New York: Semiotext Books.

FREIRE, P., 1972. *Pedagogy of the oppressed*. London: Penguin.

GRAMSCI, A., 1971. *The prison notebooks*. London: Lawrence and Wishart.

HAMALAINEN, J., 2003. The concept of social pedagogy in the field of social work. *Journal of social work*, 3(1), 70-80. https://doi.org/10.1177/1468017303003001005

HATTON, K., 2013. *Social pedagogy in the UK: Theory and practice*. Lyme Regis: Russell House Publishing.

HATTON, K., 2015. *New directions in social work practice*, 2nd ed. London: Learning Matters/ Sage.

HATTON, K., 2017. A critical examination of the knowledge contribution service user and carer involvement brings to social work education. *Social work education*, 36(2), 154-171. https://doi.org/10.1080/02615479.2016.1254769

HATTON, K., 2020. A new framework for creativity in social pedagogy. *International journal of social pedagogy*, 9(1), 16. https://doi.org/10.14324/111.444.ijsp.2020.v9.x.016

HILL COLLINS, P. and S. BILGE, 2016. *Intersectionality*. Cambridge: Polity.

HUMPHREYS, C., 2005. Service user involvement in social work education: A case example. *Social work education*, 24, 797-803. https://doi.org/10.1080/02615470500238710

IRVINE, J., J. MOLYNEUX and M. GILLMAN, 2015. Providing a link with the real world: Learning from the student experience of service user and carer involvement in social work education. *Social work education*, 34, 138-150. https://doi.org/10.1080/02615479.2014.957178

JORDAN, B. and M. DRAKEFORD, 2012. *Social work and social policy under austerity*. Basingstoke: Palgrave Macmillan.

McLAUGHLIN, H., 2009. 'What's in a name': Client, patient, customer, consumer, expert by experience, service user: What's next?'. *The British journal of social work*, 39(6), 1101-1117. https://doi.org/10.1093/bjsw/bcm155

SHAKESPEARE, T., 2013. *Disability rights and wrongs revisited*. London, Routledge.

SKOURA-KIRK, E., *et al*., 2013. Mark my words! Service user and carer involvement in social work academic assessment. *Social work education*, 32, 560-575. https://doi.org/10.1080/02615 479.2012.690388

SOCIAL CARE INSTITUTE FOR EXCELLENCE, 2011. *What is personalisation?* [viewed 15 December 2022]. Available from: www.scie.org.uk/personalisation/introduction/what-is

SOCIAL CARE INSTITUTE FOR EXCELLENCE, 2022. *Co-production: What it is and how to do it* [viewed 15 December 2022]. Available from: www.scie.org.uk/co-production/what-how

TEW, J., 2006. Understanding power and powerlessness: Towards a framework for emancipatory practice in social work. *Journal of social work*, 6, 33-51. https://doi.org/10.1177/146801730 6062222

VYGOTSKY, L., 2004. Imagination and creativity in childhood. *Journal of Russian and East European psychology*, 42, 7-97. https://doi.org/10.1080/10610405.2004.11059210

WATERSON, J. and K. MORRIS, 2005. Training in 'social' work: Exploring issues of involving users in teaching on social work degree programmes. *Social work education*, 24, 653-675. https://doi.org/10.1080/02615470500185093

WEBBER, M. and K. ROBINSON, 2012. The meaningful involvement of service users and carers in advanced-level post-qualifying social work education: A qualitative study. *British journal of social work*, 42, 1256-1274. https://doi.org/10.1093/bjsw/bcr141

11 Ethics and ethical dilemmas in health and social care

Gemma Burley and Lisa Arai

Box 11.1: Contents

- Introduction
- What does 'ethics' mean?
- Ethics: Do they matter?
- Main ethical theories and frameworks
- Ethical dilemmas in health and social care
- Living the ethical life

Box 11.2: Learning outcomes

By the end of this chapter, you should be able to

- Explain what 'ethics' means
- Discuss the main ethical theories and principles
- Identify biomedical ethical principles
- Reflect on the importance of good ethical conduct in health and social care.

Box 11.3: Keywords

- Informed consent
- Autonomy
- Virtue ethics
- Utilitarianism
- Biomedical ethics
- Principalism
- Ethical dilemmas

DOI: 10.4324/9781003198338-14

Introduction

The aim of this chapter is to examine ethical concepts and theories and explore ethical dilemmas in health and social care (H&SC). You will learn what the word 'ethics' means and consider why ethical practice is so important. We will also briefly examine how people can engage in ethical behaviour every day.

Students who are already in practice are likely to have encountered ethical dilemmas in their workplace, so some of the contents of this chapter will have special resonance. Readers who are not practitioners may have experienced ethical dilemmas in other, non-H&SC, spheres. Indeed, ethical dilemmas can arise in all settings and can be frequent and seemingly intractable (or 'thorny') in nature. However, the difficulties inherent in resolving ethical dilemmas do not remove the need to attempt to do so. This is especially important for H&SC workers who are often supporting people when they are at their most vulnerable, when they are in pain, distress or bereaved.

What does 'ethics' mean?

> Activity 11.1: What does 'ethics' mean?
>
> Ethics was mentioned in chapter 3. Do you know what this term means? Make a note of your answer.

Ethics is concerned with notions of right and wrong; it's about 'doing the right thing'. Ethics are strongly related to values and morals; values refer to the beliefs that we consider important and that influence our actions, and morals are the sets of rules governing how people live in the society and vary from one place to another and from one period to another.

Ethical theories and principles can be used to help H&SC practitioners to decide on the best course of action when faced with a dilemma such as whether it's permissible to breach patient confidentiality when there is a risk to life or well-being or where a patient refuses necessary treatment.

Autonomy and informed consent

Treatment refusal is related to the central (and, arguably the most important) ethical concept of autonomy; the right of individuals to decide what happens to them, to have control over their own bodies. The challenges around safeguarding patient autonomy can be considerable, and most H&SC workers are likely to experience them at some point in their career. Ulrich *et al.*'s (2010) analysis of data collected from a large sample of US nurses found that the most common (and stressful) ethical patient care dilemmas included the challenges of protecting patients' rights, safeguarding autonomy and securing informed consent. Informed consent means that patients and service users are given all necessary information before deciding on what treatment they will receive. The British Medical Association (2020) notes that, in medical care:

... autonomy is usually expressed as the right of competent adults to make informed decisions about their own medical care. The principle underlies the requirement to seek the consent or informed agreement of the patient before any investigation or treatment takes place. The principle is perhaps seen at its most forcible when patients exercise their autonomy by refusing life-sustaining treatment.

Ulrich *et al.* (2010) advise that the ethical challenges faced by nurses seeking informed consent and ensuring autonomy, as well as other ethical dilemmas, will become more frequent as practitioners deal with the consequences of looking after chronically ill patients in an ageing society.

Varkey (2021) observes that respecting the principle of autonomy obliges the physician to disclose medical information and treatment options that are necessary for the patient to exercise self-determination. What does this concept mean in practice? See Panels 11.1 and 11.2 below.

Panel 11.1: Informed consent in health and social care practice in the Nursing and Midwifery Council's Code of Practice

The Nursing and Midwifery Council's Code of Practice stipulates that, to act in the best interests of people at all times, nurses, midwives and nursing associates must: '...make sure that you get proper informed consent and document it before carrying out any action' (Nursing and Midwifery Council 2018, p.7).

The National Health Service (NHS) refers to 'consent to treatment'. This means: '... a person must give permission before they receive any type of medical treatment, test or examination...Consent from a patient is needed regardless of the procedure, whether it's a physical examination, organ donation or something else'. Moreover, for consent to be valid, it must be informed'. 'Informed', here, means that the patient must be given information about what the treatment involves, and the benefits and risks associated with the treatment as well as whether or not there are alternative treatments. Patients should also be told what will happen if treatment does not go ahead (NHS 2019).

Sometimes, it's difficult to obtain informed consent. A patient may lack capacity, for example, and may not able to make decisions for themselves about their care. If this is the case, the *Mental Capacity Act (2005)* can be used.

There may be differences in legal jurisdictions.

Panel 11.2: The General Medical Council's seven principles of decision making and consent

1. All patients have the right to be involved in decisions about their treatment and should be supported to make informed decisions where they are able to do so
2. Decision making is an ongoing process involving dialogue between the professional(s) and the patient

3. All patients have the right to be listened to and to be given the information they need to decide about their treatment
4. Doctors must establish what's important to patients so that they can share information about the benefits and harms of treatment options
5. Doctors must presume that all adult patients have the capacity to make decisions about their treatment. A patient can be judged to lack capacity after only appropriate assessment
6. The choice of treatment for patients lacking capacity must benefit them, and decisions should be made in consultation with their advocates
7. Patients whose right to consent is affected by law should be supported to be involved in the decision-making process and to exercise choice where possible

Adapted from: General Medical Council (2020).

What are the other important ethical principles in H&SC practice?

Other ethical principles that H&SC workers need to be mindful of when treating patients or when working with service users include:

• Confidentiality and privacy: the Nursing and Midwifery Council Code (2018) states that nurses, midwives and nursing associates must respect people's right to privacy and people are informed about how and why information is used and shared by those who will be providing care. Information can be shared with others when the interests of patient safety and public protection override the need for confidentiality
• Anti-discriminatory practice: Social Care Institute for Excellence (2020) observe that anti-discriminatory practice is '...fundamental to the ethical basis of care provision and critical to the protection of people's dignity' and cite the *Equality Act (2010) as* important legislation in protecting people receiving care as well as the workers providing it from being treated unfairly
• Dignity and respect: Article I of the Universal Declaration of Human Rights (United Nations 1948) states that: 'All human beings are born free and equal in dignity and rights'. 'Dignity' is not easy to define but, in essence, it's about the right to be treated with respect. The code of the International Council of Nurses' (International Council of Nurses 2021) observes that 'Inherent in nursing is a respect for human rights, includingcultural rights, the right to life and choice, the right to dignity and to be treated with respect' (p.2).

Ethics: do they matter?

Activity 11.2: Do ethics matter?

Before we examine the main ethical theories, think about why this concept is so important. Do ethics matter? Can you think of situations or examples where there has been a breach of ethics? What happened and why?

Hopefully, you do think that ethics and ethical principles are important. You'd probably wouldn't read this book if you were the kind of person who thought this wasn't true. Practitioner readers wouldn't have a very long or fruitful career in H&SC if they didn't believe in the importance of ethical behaviour.

However, even in H&SC settings where the general expectation is that sound ethical practice is paramount, there have been some high-profile scandals where practitioners have behaved unethically. We will look at one of the examples now.

Mid Staffordshire ('Mid Staffs') National Health Service Foundation Trust

Between 400 and 1,200 patients died as a result of poor care over the 4-year period from 2005 to 2009 at Stafford Hospital in Staffordshire. In 2007, the NHS care regulator noted the unusually high death rates at the hospital, and concerns quickly mounted about care at the Trust. The report of the Mid Staffordshire NHS Foundation Trust Public Inquiry (Francis 2013) noted that the inquiry heard 'harrowing' stories from patients and their families about the care at the Trust and that many of the cases were related to basic patient care. The Inquiry referred to:

- Patients left in excrement in soiled bed clothes for long periods
- Assistance with feeding not provided for patients who needed feeding support
- Water left out of patients' reach
- Patients not assisted in their toileting
- A general denial of privacy and dignity, even in death
- The callous treatment of patients by staff (p.19)

One of the many recommendations made after the scandal included the requirement for a greater focus on compassion among care workers. This led to the development of a document called 'Compassion in Practice', which described the six 'Cs' of nursing (care, compassion, courage, communication, commitment and competence) (Bivins, Tierney and Seers 2017).

Panel 11.3: Read more about the Mid Staffs hospital scandal

Read more about the Mid Staffs scandal at: www.theguardian.com/society/2013/feb/06/mid-staffs-hospital-scandal-guide#107
  and
  https://assets.publishing.service.gov.uk/government/uploads/system/uploads/attachment_data/file/279124/0947.pdf
  www.nuffieldtrust.org.uk/media/robert-francis-insights-into-the-mid-staffordshire-inquiry

---

Thus far, we have defined ethics, discussed some key ethical principles and considered why ethics is important in H&SC. We will now examine some ethical theories and frameworks. Ethics have been studied since at least the time of the ancient Greeks, and there are many theoretical perspectives and concepts to draw on. However, no one theory can provide an adequate framework for all ethical decisions.

Main ethical theories and frameworks

Aristotelian ethics

Aristotle (384–322 BC) believed that the key to ethical behaviour lies within the person himself or herself; good people make good ethical decisions. For this reason, Aristotelian ethics is also called 'virtue ethics', which is a:

> …character-based approach to morality assumes that we acquire virtue through practice. By practicing being honest, brave, just, generous, and so on, a person develops an honourable and moral character. According to Aristotle, by honing virtuous habits, people will likely make the right choice when faced with ethical challenges (McCombs School of Business 2022).

Consequentialism

'Consequentialism' refers to ethical frameworks that judge actions in terms of the outcome rather than the actions ('the ends justify the means'). Utilitarianism is a form of consequentialism. Utilitarianists are concerned only with outcomes and with decisions, which minimise harm and maximise benefits to the greatest number of people ('the greatest happiness to the greatest number'). From a utilitarian perspective, some harmful actions to individuals are acceptable and justifiable for an overall net benefit to the larger population (Vearrier and Henderson 2021).

Panel 11.4: Famous utilitarianists

Important utilitarians were Jeremy Bentham (1748–1832) and John Stuart Mill (1808–73). Both were English philosophers who espoused the idea that the greatest happiness should derive to the greatest number.

Jeremy Bentham was a noted eccentric who stipulated that his body be preserved after his death and left elaborate instructions on how this was to be done. You can see his preserved body (minus the head) on display in University College, London. See Figure 11.1.

Deontology

Immanuel Kant (1724–1804) is associated with this philosophical tradition. Kant viewed ethical behaviour as arising from a sense of 'doing one's duty' and argued that some ethical requirements are unconditional and universal regardless of consequences. At the heart of this school of thought is Kant's 'categorical imperative': a universal ethical principle that holds that you should respect others' humanity and that you should act only in accordance with universal rules (Jankowiak 2022). Deontology is simple to apply, as it requires that people:

> …follow the rules and do their duty. This approach tends to fit well with our natural intuition about what is or isn't ethical. Unlike consequentialism, which judges actions

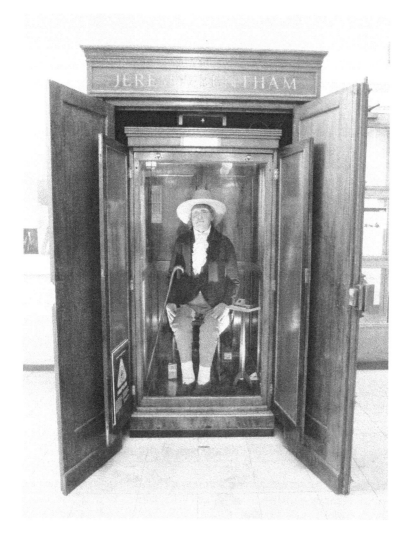

Figure 11.1 Jeremy Bentham's preserved body

by their results, deontology doesn't require weighing the costs and benefits of a situation. This avoids subjectivity and uncertainty because you have to follow only set rules. Despite its strengths, rigidly following deontology can produce results that many people find unacceptable (https://ethicsunwrapped.utexas.edu/glossary/deontology)

The Georgetown Mantra and principalism

The frameworks described above were not created specially with health or medical care in mind and may be of limited use in H&SC settings where workers need to make ethical decisions often under pressure and in busy and challenging conditions. The seminal work by Beauchamp and Childress (1985) on biomedical ethical principles was developed specifically to be used in healthcare settings. The four principles are:

- Respect for autonomy: this has been already explored earlier. This is the need to '... respect the decision-making capacities of autonomous persons' (Beauchamp 2003, p.269)
- Non-maleficence: Not causing harm (physical, emotional, etc.) to people
- Beneficence: This is the requirement to provide benefits for people, and to balance benefits against risks
- Justice: Beauchamp (2003) defines this as: 'Obligations of fairness in the distribution of benefits and risks (p.269).

These principles are called the 'Georgetown mantra' because they grew out of work conducted at Georgetown University in the United States of America (USA) and are the main elements of what's called 'principalism'.

Ethical dilemmas in Health and Social Care

The Oxford Dictionary defines an ethical dilemma as: 'a situation in which a difficult choice has to be made between two courses of action, either of which entails transgressing a moral principle'.

H&SC practitioners often have to make complex decisions regarding patient care, and the best course of action is not always clear. An example often seen in ethical debates is in respect of the withdrawal of life-sustaining treatment. The withdrawal of such treatment revolves around the removal or cessation of treatment prolonging a patient's life and can involve the removal of equipment such as ventilators or cessation of nutritional/fluid support, which will, ultimately, result in the patient's death. The decision to withdraw treatment is usually made by a variety of people, including clinicians, the patient and family members, all of whom must consider the moral and clinical implications of the decision. However, it is also not uncommon in healthcare for people to hold opposing opinions so that family members don't always agree with clinical decisions, for example, or different clinicians may hold different views about the correct course of action. This can cause further practical ethical dilemmas as it's not always clear what action to take.

While ethical dilemmas in H&SC have always been present, the emergence of social media and news coverage has increased the general public's awareness of some of these dilemmas.

Activity 11.3: Can you think of any recent ethical health-related dilemmas?

The withdrawal of life-sustaining treatment can be an emotive topic, and there have been several high-profile cases seen in the media, especially when there has been a disagreement between clinicians and family members. Can you think of any dilemmas you have seen over the last few years?

Recent court cases that you might have been aware of include those of Archie Battersbee (*Barts Health NHS Trust v Dance and Battersbee [2022] EWHC 1435 (Fam)* 2022) and

Alfie Evans (*Alder Hey Children's NHS Foundation Trust v Evans and Anor [2018] EWHC 308 (Fam)* 2018). These are cases where families disagreed with medical professionals' decision to remove life-sustaining treatment. Both cases included the hospital trust applying to the High Court to allow clinicians to remove treatment against the families' wishes (the trusts' cases were upheld but only after several appeals by the families of both children). These cases gained large news and social media coverage, nationally and globally, and raised strong opinions on both sides of the decision.

As highlighted in the above cases, UK law has an important role to play in ethical dilemmas in healthcare. Clinicians are governed by their own professional regulations (General Medical Council, Nursing and Midwifery Council, etc.) and also by their own country's laws. The use of UK legislation is an important part of ethical dilemmas and decision-making processes. However, while generally seen as a protective part of ethical dilemmas (clinicians must practise within the law), the impact of legislation on healthcare can lead to negative clinical outcomes and to more ethical and moral dilemmas for patients and clinicians.

An example of this can be seen in respect of abortion. This is a controversial topic characterised by often strong opposing viewpoints about the right of women to access legal abortion. The ongoing ethical debate around abortion access centres on the rights of the mother and rights of the unborn foetus. When does a foetus have rights? At the time of conception? Once the pregnancy becomes viable?

These questions govern the legal and ethical availability of safe abortion care. In England, Scotland and Wales, women have the legal right to have an abortion before the 24th week of pregnancy under the *Abortion Act (1967)*. However, abortion access differs across the globe, with some countries restricting women's right to choose an abortion access by imposing limits on when an abortion can take place or under what circumstances. Some countries do not allow it under any circumstance.

Abortion access was propelled into the forefront of political discussion in 2022 after the supreme court overruled Roe v. Wade (Justia US Supreme Court 1973) in the USA. This removed the accepted understanding that abortion was a constitutional right for American citizens and, after the overturning of Roe v. Wade, individual states could regulate citizens' rights to abortion access. This resulted in 11 of 50 states imposing a near-total ban on abortions (Abortion Finder 2022).

An important issue to consider in terms of ethical debates about access to abortion is the implications to women's health where safe abortion care is not provided. Stevenson (2021) estimated that a ban on abortion in the USA could result in a 21% increase in pregnancy mortality. The World Health Organization (2020) regards abortion care as an essential healthcare service and highlights the negative implications of a lack of access to safe abortion care: 'unsafe abortion is a leading—but preventable—cause of maternal deaths and morbidities. It can lead to physical and mental health complications and social and financial burdens for women, communities and healthcare systems' (World Health Organization 2021).

The death of Savita Halappanavar highlighted the possible consequences to patients' health when they are denied access to safe abortion care (McDonnell and Murphy 2019). Savita died in Ireland in 2012, after being admitted to hospital with an incomplete miscarriage. Because of the unclear laws regarding abortion access in Ireland at that time, Savita was denied an abortion, she later developed sepsis and died from a cardiac arrest on 28 October 2012, which was 7 days after being admitted to the hospital (Arulkumaran 2013). This case became known worldwide and highlighted the debate on the ethical dilemma of abortion care in Ireland and was a key force in the eventual repeal of Ireland's Eight Amendment that allowed safe access to abortion care in Ireland (Drążkiewicz and Strong 2020).

Living the ethical life

Our examination of ethics has been highly theoretical thus far. We have defined ethics, considered why it's important, discussed various ethical theories and frameworks and examined some contemporary ethical dilemmas. What does all of these mean for everyday life? How can people—H&SC workers and others—behave in ethical ways in everyday life?

Shanks (1995) observes that most people would like to live an ethical life but are likely to encounter 'everyday stumbling blocks' to ethical behaviour. These include beliefs that their own (small) effort won't make a difference, that it might affect what people think of them, that it's difficult to know the right thing to do and that it may hurt their career. Shanks asks us to consider how we'd respond if our children were the ones making excuses like this for their behaviour. In short, he writes, people need a systematic way to live an ethical life.

To do this, Shanks suggests that people ask themselves five questions every day. These are:

1. *Did I practise any virtues today?* Did I show integrity, trustworthiness, honesty, compassion or any of the other virtues I was taught as a child?
2. *Did I do more good than harm today?* Or did I try to? What are the short- and long-term consequences of my actions?
3. *Did I treat people with dignity and respect today?* How did my actions respect the moral rights and dignity to which every person is entitled?
4. *Was I fair and just today?* Did I treat each person the same unless there was some reason to treat him or her differently?
5. *Was my community better because I was in it?* Was I better because I was in my community?

Activity 11.4: What do you think of these five questions?

What do you think of these five questions? Could asking yourself questions like these guide you in your everyday life? Can you think of any other questions you might ask yourself?

Summary

In this chapter, we explored ethics, ethical principles and frameworks, ethical dilemmas and everyday ethical behaviour. The Mid Staffordshire ('Mid Staffs') NHS Foundation Trust scandal—a high-profile example of a breach of clinical care that contributed to the deaths of many patients and that was the subject of several government inquiries—was discussed. Some general ethical theories and frameworks, such as consequentialism and deontology, were described. An ethical framework developed specifically for healthcare settings (principalism) was examined. This contains four main elements: autonomy, non-maleficence, beneficence and justice. A framework for living an ethical life was also briefly considered. This recommends that people ask themselves five questions every day to ascertain to what extent they are living an ethical life.

You may find, as a result of reading the numerous theories and frameworks, that you are more confused than ever about how to resolve an issue or problem. It's often the case that it's not easy to know how to resolve a dilemma and, in fact, there often is no one 'right' way to do so. This does not remove the need to practise ethical conduct in everyday life, especially for H&SC workers dealing with people when they are at their most vulnerable.

Box 11.4: Key learning points

- Ethics is about 'doing the right thing'
- Autonomy—the right to make your own decisions about what happens to you and what treatment you receive—is a central ethical principle
- Ethical behaviour in health and social care is important to the provision of safe, effective clinical care
- There are many ethical theories and frameworks to draw on when seeking to resolve ethical dilemmas
- Principalism is an ethical framework designed specifically for healthcare workers
- It's important to pay attention to everyday ethical behaviour.

References

ABORTION FINDER, 2022. *State-by-state guide* [viewed 11/9/22]. Available from: www.abortionfinder.org/abortion-guides-by-state

ALDER HEY CHILDREN'S NHS FOUNDATION TRUST V EVANS and ANOR [2018] EWHC 308 (Fam), 2018.

ARULKUMARAN, S., 2013. *Investigation of incident 50278 from time of patient's self referral to hospital on the 21st of October 2012 to the patient's death on the 28th of October, 2012. Health Service Executive* [viewed 11 September 2022]. Available from: http://hdl.handle.net/10147/293964

BARTS HEALTH NHS TRUST V DANCE and BATTERSBEE [2022] EWHC 1435 (Fam), 2022. www.judiciary.uk/wp-content/uploads/2022/07/Archie-Batteresbee-judgment-2-1.pdf

BEAUCHAMP, T., 2003. Methods and principles in biomedical ethics. *Journal of medical ethics*, 29, 269–274. https://doi.org/10.1136/jme.29.5.269

BEAUCHAMP, T. L. and J. F. CHILDRESS, 1985. *Principles of biomedical ethics*. USA: Oxford University Press.

BIVINS, R., S. TIERNEY and K. SEERS, 2017. Compassionate care: Not easy, not free, not only nurses. *BMJ quality and safety*, 26, 1023-1026. https://doi.org/10.1136/bmjqs-2017-007005

BRITISH MEDICAL ASSOCIATION, 2020. *Ethics toolkit for medical students*. London: BMA.

DRĄŻKIEWICZ, E. and T. STRONG, 2020. Repealing Ireland's Eighth Amendment: Abortion rights and democracy today. *Social anthropology*, 28(3), 561-566. https://doi.org/10.1111/1469-8676.12914

FRANCIS, R., 2013. *Report of the Mid Staffordshire NHS Foundation Trust Public Inquiry. Volume 1: Analysis of evidence and lessons learned (part 1)* [viewed 31 December 2022].

Available from: https://assets.publishing.service.gov.uk/government/uploads/system/uploads/atta chment_data/file/279115/0898_i.pdf

GENERAL MEDICAL COUNCIL, 2020. *Guidance on professional standards and ethics for doctors: Decision making and consent.* London: GMC.

INTERNATIONAL COUNCIL OF NURSES, 2021. *The ICN code of ethics for nurses.* Geneva, Switzerland: ICN.

JANKOWIAK, T., 2022. *Immanuel Kant* [viewed 31 December 2022]. The Internet Encyclopedia of Philosophy (IEP). Available from: https://iep.utm.edu/kantview/

JUSTIA US SUPREME COURT, 1973. *Roe v Wade, 410 U.S. 113 (1973)* [viewed 31 December 2022]. Available from: https://supreme.justia.com/cases/federal/us/410/113/

MCCOMBS SCHOOL OF BUSINESS, 2022. *Virtue ethics* [viewed 15 December 2022]. *Austin, Texas: McCombs School of Business, the University of Texas at Austin.* Available from: https://ethicsunwrapped.utexas.edu/glossary/virtue-ethics

MCDONNELL, O. and P. MURPHY, 2019. Mediating abortion politics in Ireland: Media framing of the death of Savita Halappanavar. *Critical discourse studies,* 16(1), 1-20. https://doi.org/10.1080/17405904.2018.1521858

NHS 2019. *Overview: Consent to treatment* [viewed: 15 July 2023]. Available from: https://www.nhs.uk/conditions/consent-to-treatment/

NURSING AND MIDWIFERY COUNCIL, 2018. *The code: Professional standards of practice and behaviour for nurses, midwives and nursing associates* [viewed 15 December 2022]. London: NMC. Available from: www.nmc.org.uk/globalassets/sitedocuments/nmc-publications/nmc-code.pdf

SHANKS, T., 1995. *Everyday ethics* [viewed 15 December 2022]. Santa Clara, CA: Markkula Center for Applied Ethics. Available from: www.scu.edu/ethics/ethics-resources/ethical-decision-making/everyday-ethics/

SOCIAL CARE INSTITUTE FOR EXCELLENCE, 2020. *Equality Act 2010* [viewed 15 December 2022]. London: Social Care Institute for Excellence. Available from: www.scie.org.uk/key-social-care-legislation/equality-act

STEVENSON, A. J., 2021. The pregnancy-related mortality impact of a total abortion ban in the United States: A research note on increased deaths due to remaining pregnant. *Demography,* 58(6), 2019-2028. https://doi.org/10.1215/00703370-9585908

ULRICH, C. M. *et al.*, 2010. Everyday ethics: ethical issues and stress in nursing practice. *Journal of advanced nursing,* 66(11), 2510-2519. https://doi.org/10.1111/j.1365-2648.2010.05425.x

UNITED NATIONS, 1948. *The universal declaration of human rights* [viewed 15 December 2022]. New York: United Nations. Available from: www.un.org/en/about-us/universal-declaration-of-human-rights

VARKEY, B., 2021. Principles of clinical ethics and their application to practice. *Medical principles and practice,* 30, 17-28. https://doi.org/10.1159/000509119

VEARRIER, L. and C. M. HENDERSON, 2021. Utilitarian principlism as a framework for crisis healthcare ethics. *HEC forum,* 33, 45-60. https://doi.org/10.1007/s10730-020-09431-7

WORLD HEALTH ORGANIZATION, 2021. *Abortion* [viewed 11 September 2022]. Available from: www.who.int/news-room/fact-sheets/detail/abortion

WORLD HEALTH ORGANIZATION, 2020. *Maintaining essential health services: Operational guidance for the COVID-19 context.* Geneva: World Health Organization.

Part 4

Improving Services, Improving Health

12 Introduction to public health and health promotion

Lisa Arai

Box 12.1: Contents

- Introduction
- What is public health?
- A brief history of public health
- Epidemiology and public health
- Intervening to promote health: Key concepts
- 21st-century public health: Your role in promoting health and well-being

---

Box 12.2: Learning outcomes

By the end of this chapter, you should be able to

- Define public health
- Describe the history of public health in the United Kingdom
- Understand how data are used in public health
- Identify key concepts in health promotion
- Consider your own role in promoting health and well-being now and in the future.

Box 12.3: Keywords

- Public health
- Health promotion
- Intervention
- Epidemiology
- Demography
- Prevalence
- Ethics
- Stewardship model
- Intervention ladder

DOI: 10.4324/9781003198338-16

Introduction

If you had asked the man or woman in the street what 'public health' means *before* the COVID-19 pandemic, it is possible that he or she wouldn't have known how to answer. The pandemic has—arguably—led to a greater, general understanding of public health (best seen in the widespread use of public health terms such as 'social distancing' and 'quarantine'). While managing viral threats is an important public health activity, public health is not solely about protecting people from infection. It is much more than this, as we shall see in this chapter where we examine contemporary public health and health promotion in the United Kingdom (UK), explore its historical development, discuss the use of public health data and consider your role (as current or future health and social care [H&SC] professionals) in promoting health and well-being.

What is public health?

Activity 12.1: Can you define public health?

Before we explore definitions of public health, can you define public health in one or two sentences?

An early definition of public health is that by the American bacteriologist, C-E. A. Winslow who wrote nearly 100 years ago that public health is:

> ...the science and art of preventing disease, prolonging life and promoting physical health and efficiency through organised community efforts for the sanitation of the environment, the control of community infections, the education of the individual in personal hygiene, the organization of medical and nursing services for early diagnosis and preventive treatment of disease and the development of the social machinery, which will ensure to every individual in the community a standard of living adequate for maintenance of health ... (Winslow 1920, p.30).

Winslow's famous definition can be compared with a contemporary one by the UK-based Faculty of Public Health (FPH), where public health is defined as:

> ... the science and art of promoting and protecting health and well-being, preventing ill-health and prolonging life through the organised efforts of the society (Faculty of Public Health 2016, p.2).

While there are differences in these definitions (Winslow's reference to 'sanitation of the environment' and education in 'personal hygiene' reflects the health threats of his age— infectious or 'communicable' diseases—diseases spread from one person to another), both definitions refer to the core public health activities of *promoting health* and *preventing ill health*. Winslow's 'social machinery' is comparable to the FPH's 'organised efforts of society' in terms of reflecting the importance of understanding how broader, societal factors influence health and well-being.

Winslow refers to medical and nursing services. What role do H&SC professionals play in public health? Public health is not about diagnosing individual patients as a general practitioner might. Instead, populations—small ones such as workers in a specific industry, or larger groups such as entire communities or even national or international populations—are the primary focus of interest in public health. The perspective adopted in public health is a 'bigger picture' one, although workers with a public health remit may find that they interact on a one-to-one interaction with individuals when, for example, promoting health.

According to Health Education England (2020), public health work is considered to fall into four 'domains':

* health improvement (health promotion)
* healthcare public health (healthcare provision)
* academic public health (developing the evidence public health practice relies on) and
* health protection (reducing the risks from infectious diseases and other emergencies)

You can see the diversity and scope of public health work in these four domains.

Activity 12.2: Watch Health Education England's short videos

Watch Health Education England's short videos describe the four domains of public health work. These are:

* What is health improvement? Watch at: https://youtube/0JPe-U4iLMA
* What is healthcare public health? Watch at: https://youtube/wJUmIksvYG0
* What is academic public health? Watch at: https://youtube/CIzSDmWUGqM
* What is health protection? Watch at: https://youtube/RgnCUrdZ688

A brief history of public health

To explore the history of public health, we will draw on Hanlon *et al.*'s (2011) analysis of public health history in the UK. These authors write that four 'waves' of public health activity from the Industrial Revolution to the present day can be discerned. For these authors, each wave is related to 'shifts in thinking about the nature of the society and health itself' (p.30).

The first wave: 19th century England

The first wave is in the 19th century and is focused on the work of great Victorian social reformers such as Edwin Chadwick and the introduction of the first public health legislation (the *Public Health Act of 1848*; UK Parliament 2022). This wave of public health activity took place against a backdrop of rapid urbanisation; the movement of people from rural locations into town and cities to work in the factories and mills of London and other cities. Conditions in the 19th century urban centres were extremely damaging to health. Streets were dirty, the water supply was unsafe and the air was badly polluted.

Most ordinary people laboured for long hours for little recompense and lived with their families in slum conditions.

Fredrick Engels, the German-born social reformer and co-founder of communism, provided a powerful account of England's slums in 'The Condition of the Working Class in England' of 1845. Writing of one London district, St Giles, he described it as:

> ...a disorderly collection of tall ...houses, with narrow, crooked, filthy streets ... here, people of the working-class only are to be seen ... The houses are occupied from cellar to garret, filthy within and without, and their appearance is such that no human being could possibly wish to live in them. But all this is nothing in comparison with the dwellings in the narrow courts and alleys between the streets, entered by covered passages between the houses, in which the filth and tottering ruin surpass all description. Scarcely, a whole window-pane can be found, the walls are crumbling, door-posts and window-frames loose and broken, doors of old boards nailed together, or altogether wanting in this thieves' quarter, where no doors are needed, there being nothing to steal. Heaps of garbage and ashes lie in all directions, and the foul liquids emptied before the doors gather in stinking pools. Here live the poorest of the poor, the worst paid workers with thieves and the victims of prostitution indiscriminately huddled together ... in the whirlpool of moral ruin, which surrounds them, sinking daily deeper, losing daily more and more of their power to resist the demoralising influence of want, filth and evil surroundings (Engels 1845/1993).

Tuberculosis, cholera and typhoid are all conditions associated with poverty and lack of access to clean water, thrived in these overcrowded and filthy conditions. Communicable diseases such as these represented the greatest threat to health, so public health reformers of the day focused their energies on provision of clean drinking water, sewerage systems and better working conditions. Two health reformers of this period, Sir Edwin Chadwick and Dr John Snow, played important public health roles in this period. See Panel 12.1.

Panel 12.1: Victorian public health reformers

Edwin Chadwick (1800–1890) argued in his 'Sanitary condition of the labouring population of Great Britain' (Chadwick 1842) that sanitation measures (potable water, sewerage systems, clean air) would help the urban poor. His campaigning work led to the *Public Health Act* of 1848. The Act established a General Board of Health, which could create local health boards. The latter had the authority to deal with the water supply, sewage and rubbish removal.

The 1848 Act established a legislative public health framework and helped lay the groundwork for future developments such as the *Public Health Act* of 1875 but was limited in that it did not compel action (UK Parliament 2022). By contrast, the 1875 Act required local authorities to make provision of clean water, refuse removal, etc. Under the 1875, all homes had to be connected to the main sewerage system (Health Foundation 2022).

Dr John Snow (1813–1858), the author of 'On the Mode of Communication of Cholera' (Snow 1849), mapped cases during a cholera outbreak in Soho (London)

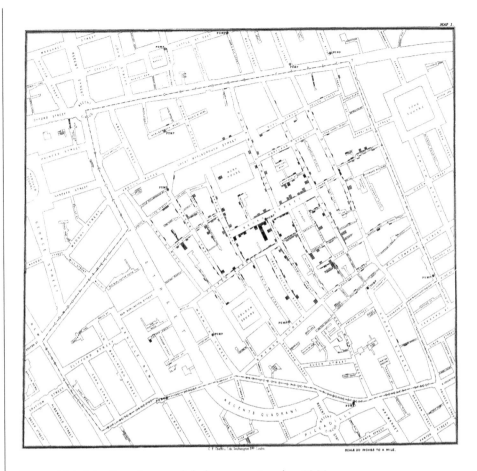

Figure 12.1 John Snow's map of cholera cases, London 1854
Creative Commons License

in 1854 (see Figure 12.1). He identified a water pump as the source of the outbreak. The handle of the pump was removed, and the outbreak came to an end. Because of his meticulous mapping of cholera cases, John Snow is considered a founding father of epidemiology.

Activity 12.3: Read John Snow's account of the cholera outbreak

Read John Snow's account of the cholera outbreak in Soho, London, 1854 at: www.bl.uk/collection-items/john-snows-account-of-the-cholera-outbreak-in-soho-london-1854

Later waves

Hanlon *et al.* describe the second 'wave' as falling in the period 1890–1950 and refer to the use of vaccines and antibiotics as evidence of: '...the rise of scientific rationalism...' (p.31). The third 'wave' was placed in the 40-year period from 1940 to 1980 in which there was increasing recognition of lifestyle-related risk factors for illness (such as those caused by smoking).

The fourth wave began in the 1960s and continues to the present day and is primarily concerned with the economic and social factors affecting health. This important strand of work has led to a large body of research on 'health inequalities'. These are '...differences in health across the population, and between different groups in the society, that are systematic, unfair and avoidable (National Institute for Care and Excellence 2023). One of the most prolific researchers working on health inequalities is Professor Sir Michael Marmot, who wrote the 'Marmot Review' in 2010 (Marmot 2010) and a later review (Marmot *et al.* 2020).

Activity 12.4: Read Michael Marmot's work

Read the executive summary of 'Fair Society Healthy Lives (The Marmot Review)' (Marmot 2010) at: www.instituteofhealthequity.org/resources-reports/fair-society-healthy-lives-the-marmot-review/fair-society-healthy-lives-exec-summary-pdf.pdf and 'Marmot Review 10 Years On' (Marmot *et al.* 2020) at: www.instituteofhealthequity.org/resources-reports/marmot-review-10-years-on/the-marmot-review-10-years-on-executive-summary.pdf
What do the authors say about progress over the 10-year period?

Hanlon *et al.* (2011) argue that we are entering a fifth public health wave that is concerned with issues such as obesity and mental health. Poor mental health, in particular, will have a profound impact on the well-being: 'Depression and anxiety are becoming a far more significant cause of disability and chronic ill health than in previous centuries...' (p.33).

Epidemiology and public health

As we have seen, public health focuses on populations (although practitioners with a health promotion remit often work one-to-one with individuals). To meet the health needs of groups of people, public health workers must understand the size and composition of the populations they are working with, as well as its social and economic characteristics. To do this, large-scale, usually quantitative (statistical) data are utilised. Where do these data come from and how are they used?

Public health is reliant on the analysis of demographic and epidemiological data. The former is the study of populations; the latter is the study of '... the distribution and determinants of health-related states or events in specified populations, and the application of this study to the control of health problems (Centers for Disease Control and Prevention 2016). The Centers for Disease Control and Prevention (2016) observe that epidemiology is often described as the 'basic science' of public health and is an integral component of public health.

Epidemiology is a highly technical discipline, one utilising a vast array of complex measures. These are used in the detection and management of diseases and conditions (this involves the use of 'surveillance'—see Panel 12.2). It is not possible here to examine these in detail. We will examine some of the most commonly used measures below.

Panel 12.2: Surveillance

Surveillance is an activity requiring high-quality, statistical data. Surveillance is: '...the ongoing systematic collection, analysis and interpretation of data, closely integrated with the timely dissemination of the resulting information to those responsible for preventing and controlling disease and injury' (Chiolero and Buckeridge 2020).

Johnson and Bovbjerg (2020) observe that the main surveillance systems are 'active' and 'passive'. In passive surveillance, health authorities passively receive reports of suspected illness, whereas in active surveillance, cases are actively sought out. These authors write that in a hypothetical outbreak of *Salmonella* associated with a restaurant, for example, epidemiologists may contact healthcare workers in the area and ask for details of patients presenting with symptoms associated with the infection.

Prevalence and incidence

Prevalence and incidence are among the most commonly used measures in public health. The prevalence of a disease or other condition is the number of people affected by the condition at a particular point in time. The incidence represents the rate of occurrence of new cases in a specific period in a population (how fast a disease is spreading or a condition is occurring in the population) (Arnold and Neill 2020).

Prevalence is usually expressed as a percentage (calculated by multiplying by 100). If the prevalence is low (because the disease or condition is rare), then it can be expressed as the number of cases per 100,000 of the population (for example, stating that there are '77 cases per 100,000 people' rather than using the prevalence rate of '0.00077').

Cases

Cases indicate people affected by the condition or disease. Public health workers sometimes refer to 'suspected' or 'probable' cases, rather than 'confirmed' cases.

In emergency situations, case definitions necessarily reflect what Tam and Haas (2016) observe is a balance between sensitivity (case definition is broad) and specificity (case definition is narrower). These authors note that:

An initial working case definition generally favours sensitivity over specificity, as the public health consequences of missing outbreak-related cases usually outweigh the resource implications of investigating cases not related to the outbreak. As the investigation develops and more information becomes available regarding the clinical and microbiological profile of the disease, the case definition will be tightened, with increasing focus on specificity (p.42).

Population at risk

Epidemiology measures disease and other outcomes in relation to what is called the 'population at risk'. The British Medical Journal (2023) defines this as:

> ... the group of people, healthy or sick, who would be counted as cases if they had the disease being studied. For example, if a general practitioner were measuring how often patients consult him about deafness, then the population at risk would comprise those people on his list ... who might see him about a hearing problem if they had one. Patients who, although still on the list, had moved to another area would not consult that doctor. They would therefore not belong to the population at risk.

The population at risk comprise the larger pool of people who are at risk of being a case or being diagnosed with the disease or condition in question. The population at risk is often defined by age and sex (only men are at risk of developing prostate cancer, for example).

Morbidity and mortality

Morbidity is defined as the state of being symptomatic of a disease or condition, whereas mortality refers to deaths caused by the condition (Hernandez and Kim 2022). The latter is usually represented by the death (or mortality) rate. This is a crude measure, as it's simply the number of deaths (numerator) over the entire population (denominator), so cannot take into account the fact that the chance of dying varies according to age, sex, etc. Therefore, the crude death rate would be high where a population is older and lower in a younger population. However, in settings where there are no age-specific or other data, it can be a useful measure. Where age-specific mortality data are available, this allows epidemiologists to calculate the mortality rate for a particular age group, like under 5s or 11- to 15-year olds, or people aged over 65 years. The denominator here is the population that falls into the specific age range.

Intervening to promote health: key concepts

Once a health problem or need is identified in a population, efforts can then be made to address or manage it. This is done through health promotion: a core public health activity and one of the domains of public health referred to earlier in this chapter.

Ottawa Charter for Health Promotion (1986)

Health promotion has, of course, a long history; Raingruber (2017) describes the ancient Greeks as one of the first civilisations to make links between health and physical and social environments and human behaviour. However, the first international health promotion conference occurred in Ottawa in 1986. This was held in response to growing international hopes for a new public health movement and led to the launch of the 'Health for all' initiative and the 'Ottawa Charter for Health Promotion' (World Health Organization 2022).

Fry and Zask (2017) maintain that the Ottawa Charter (where health promotion was defined as: 'the process of enabling people to increase control over, and to improve their health') continues to be significant in health promotion strategies many decades later. The three strategies defined in the Charter (advocacy for favourable conditions for health, enabling people to reach their full health potential and mediation between diverse societal interests for health promotion) and five areas of action (developing healthy public policy, creation of environments to improve living and working conditions, strengthening of community action, developing people's personal skills through health education and reorienting health services towards health promotion) point to its 'conceptual clarity and wide applicability…and relevance to contemporary issues' (p.902).

The Ottawa Charter informs and inspires health promotion activities to this day, although there has been a significant shift in how health promotion is conceptualised. As Raingruber (2017) says, contemporary health promotion is no longer seen as an activity where healthcare professionals educate individuals about their health; ordinary people are now likely to be actively involved in health promotion decision-making, programme design and implementation.

What are the steps in health promotion design and implementation? What kinds of issues do health promoters need to consider when designing programmes? This is a vast and complex area, and there is not the space here to fully consider it. However, we will briefly consider some key concepts below.

Key health promotion concepts

Intervention

Health promotion activities typically include the implementation of 'interventions'. These can be defined as:

> … any activity undertaken with the objective of improving human health by preventing disease, by curing or reducing the severity or duration of an existing disease, or by restoring function lost through disease or injury (Smith, Morrow and Ross 2015, p.6).

Interventions (which can also be called 'programmes' or 'initiatives') vary in size, scale and scope. Some can be small-scale (a leaflet provided by a nurse) or larger scale (like a national programme aimed at preventing child obesity). Some interventions run as a 'one-off' initiative; others are longer-term and can run for years (like the FAST programme to raise awareness of the need to respond quickly to stroke, which has been running in England since 2009; Department of Health 2009).

Intervention designers consider all aspects of the intervention—the type of intervention (for example, an exercise-based programme to reduce child obesity, a social media campaign to raise awareness of bowel cancer screening), the type of people whom it will target (women at risk of heart disease, men at risk of prostate cancer), place where it will be delivered (in primary care settings, through mainstream media) and how frequently it will be delivered (twice a week, ongoing).

In addition, as most public health interventions attempt to change behaviour, intervention developers might draw on a theory of behaviour change such as the stages of change model (Prochaska and DiClemente 1984).

Activity 12.5: The stages of change theory

The stages of change framework (also called the Transtheoretical Model) grew out of the research by Prochaska and DiClemente from the 1970s on. The model has six stages. These are:

1. Precontemplation: no intention to act
2. Contemplation: intention to change behaviour within the next 6 months
3. Preparation: preparation for taking action within the next 30 days
4. Action: actions have been taken to change the behaviour
5. Maintenance: actions are sustained for at least 6 months
6. Termination: no desire to return to unhealthy behaviours

The originators of this theory also referred to the possibility of relapse, although this was not conceived of as a stage.

What do you think of this model? Can you think of an example of a health behaviour (such as smoking cessation, for example) that this theory can be applied to?

Designers of public health interventions might also draw on other theories, such as *Nudge*. This was developed by two US-based behavioural economists (Thaler and Sunstein 2008) and encourages behavioural change through changes to the environment and provision of incentives (see also chapter 13).

Social determinants of health

The role of the social (or wider) determinants of health should always be considered when designing an intervention, especially where behaviour change is a stated outcome. What are these? These are: '...the conditions in which people are born, grow, live, work and age and inequities in power, money and resources' (Marmot 2020, p.5).

Panel 12.3: The social determinants of health

Learn more about this important concept by visiting the written (Bibby 2018) and video resources developed by the Health Foundation at: www.health.org.uk/publi cations/what-makes-us-healthy

---

Ethical issues

The designers of interventions must also consider ethical issues when creating health promotion initiatives. We explored ethics in chapter 11; this is about 'doing the right thing' and ensuring that people are not harmed by their participation in research or other activities. In chapter 11, we also considered the importance of securing informed consent from individuals because their autonomy (their right to decide what happens to then) is paramount.

Respecting autonomy and seeking consent are comparatively straightforward in most clinical settings because healthcare workers treat patients one-to-one. However, public health campaigns are often aimed at entire populations. A recent example of this can be seen in the UK and other governments' efforts to deal with COVID-19. These involved information and awareness raising campaigns and implementation of social distancing and lockdown under threat of legal sanction. Under circumstances where there is a serious threat to health, it's impossible for governments to secure informed consent from everyone in the population in terms of participation in these activities. Therefore, in public health, individual autonomy is balanced with a broader requirement to prevent harm and protect health. How can health promotion designers ensure that, where informed consent cannot be secured because interventions are aimed at entire communities or populations, their efforts are ethical?

Frameworks have been developed to help health promoters do this. Among the most significant of these frameworks is that created by the Nuffield Council on Bioethics. The Council developed the World Health Organization's (World Health Organization 2000) 'stewardship model' (Nuffield Council on Bioethics 2007). According to the Council, the concept of 'stewardship': '… is intended to convey that liberal states have a duty to look after … needs of people individually and collectively. It emphasises the obligation of states to provide conditions that allow people to be healthy… (Nuffield Council on Bioethics 2007, p.16-17).

Public health programmes implemented in a stewardship-guided state should attempt to reduce ill health through the implementation of regulations around, for example, provision of clean air and water, should pay especial attention to children's health and those who are deemed vulnerable and should aim to reduce health inequalities. Importantly public health programmes should *not* coerce adults to lead healthy lives, should minimise interventions introduced without individual consent or without 'procedural justice arrangements (such as democratic decision-making procedures), which provide adequate mandate' (p.17) and should minimise interventions considered to be intrusive or which conflict with personal values.

How can public health programme designers in a stewardship-guided state abide by these stipulations? When is it right to intervene and when is it not? Are there situations when more coercive interventions (such as those we saw in relation to COVID-19) are justified? The Nuffield Council on Bioethics refers to 'proportionality' in these matters and created the 'intervention ladder' to guide decision-making around the acceptability and justification of public health policies.

The least intrusive step at the bottom of the ladder is to do nothing and the most intrusive one is to restrict individual liberties by removing choice altogether. The Council writes that:

…the higher the rung on the ladder at which the policy maker intervenes, the stronger the justification has to be. A more intrusive policy initiative is likely to be publicly acceptable only if there is a clear indication that it will produce the desired effect, and that this can be weighed favourably against any loss of liberty that may result (p.18).

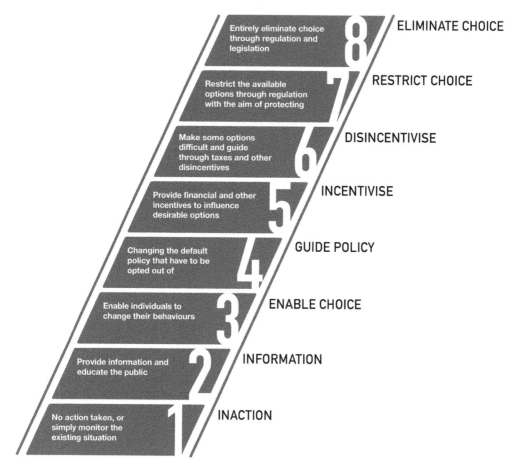

Figure 12.2 Interventions: From 'Eliminate choice' to 'Do nothing'
Image credit: Tamsin Arai Drake, adapted from: Nuffield Council on Bioethics (2007)

The ladder reflects the tensions between 'laissez-faire' approaches, which see health as the concern of the individual and not the state, and 'nanny state' ones, which advocate for the role of the state in individual health by, for example, taxing substances such as alcohol, or restricting the conditions under which some behaviours (such as smoking) can be engaged in (Thaler and Sunstein 2008).

21st-century public health: your role in promoting health and well-being

H&SC practitioners have an important role in promoting health. The Nursing and Midwifery Council's Code for nurses, midwives and nursing associates states that practitioners must ensure patients' physical, social and psychological needs are assessed and responded to and that, to achieve this, they must '…pay special attention to promoting well-being, preventing ill health and meeting the changing health and care needs of people during all stages of life' (NMC 2018, p.7). Similarly, healthcare assistant practitioner standards stipulate that, to develop skills in provision of person-centred care, apprentices should: 'promote[s] and understand[s] the impact of effective health promotion, empowering, healthy lifestyles such as movement and nutrition and fluid balance' (Institute for Apprenticeships and Technical Education 2021).

To meet the health needs of contemporary and future patients and service users, H&SC workers should stay up to date with trends and developments in population health, and those training such workers must ensure that their education includes consideration of health needs of future populations. We touched on this above when we discussed 'waves' in public health and the possibility of a fifth public health wave. What are the public health issues of the future? How can H&SC professionals be prepared for these?

Activity 12.6: What do you think will be the public health issues of the future? How can you prepare for these?

Spend a few minutes thinking about the public health issues of the future. What do you think these might be? How can you ensure you are prepared to meet the health needs of the people you care for now and in the future?

For Activity 12.6, you might have written down that the challenges presented by an ageing society will increase and this may lead to additional pressure on H&SC services. You might have noted that rates of overweight and obesity in adults and children are likely to increase, or that mental health will continue to be a concern with increasing rates of depression and anxiety. You may believe that patients and service users will engage with the care system and with their own health through the greater use of technology (in fact, technology-facilitated self-management of health is very much a contemporary phenomenon, as can be seen in the popularity of 'wearables' such as FITBIT (Dunn, Runge and Synder 2018).

One public health challenge of the near future is likely to be around the health impacts of climate change. Some of these may arise a result of extreme weather conditions (for example, the heatwaves and floods associated with global warming), and some may occur as a result of the emergence of novel infectious diseases (COVID-19 is the most recent example of this). These kinds of macro-level, environmental challenges need to be addressed by national and international governments if the health impacts on populations are to be effectively managed.

Activity 12.7: Read about the BRACE framework

The Centers for Disease Control and Prevention developed the 'Building resilience against climate effects' (BRACE) framework, to help communities prepare for the health impacts of climate change (Centers for Disease Control and Prevention 2022). Read about the framework at: www.cdc.gov/climateandhealth/BRACE.htm

Summary

This chapter defined public health, considered its history and discussed the use of epidemiological and demographic data in public health. Public health's preventative orientation is different from that of clinical healthcare, where the primary focus is on the treatment of already-diagnosed conditions. Health promotion can help in the prevention of ill health; we considered various aspects of health promotion here, including the ethical challenges raised by promoting health. As a population-related science, public health is interested in the diverse, societal-level factors affecting health and is especially mindful of the role of the social or wider determinants of health (the social and economic factors influencing health) on people's well-being. H&SC workers face many challenges addressing the health needs of contemporary populations. Many of these challenges are likely to intensify in the near future, and it's important that practitioners are prepared to deal with such scenarios.

Box 12.4: Key learning points

- Public health is concerned with promoting health and well-being and preventing ill health
- The modern public health system in the UK dates to the early 19th century and the creation of the *Public Health Act* (1848)
- Epidemiological and demographic data are essential in public health; understanding populations is key to public health practice
- Health promotion interventions vary in size, scale and scope and often utilise behavioural change theory
- Understanding the role of the wider or social determinants of health is essential to health promotion
- Health and social care practitioners have an important role in promoting health.

References

ARNOLD, S. and C. NEILL, 2020. *Incidence vs prevalence and the epidemiologist's bathtub* [viewed 4 January 2023]. Available from: www.publichealth.hscni.net/node/5277

BIBBY, J., 2018. *What makes us healthy? An introduction to the social determinants of health* [viewed 7 January 2023]. Available from: www.health.org.uk/publications/what-makes-us-healthy

BRITISH MEDICAL JOURNAL, 2023. *Chapter 1. What is epidemiology?* [viewed 4 January 2023]. Available from: www.bmj.com/about-bmj/resources-readers/publications/epidemiology-uninitia ted/1-what-epidemiology

CENTERS FOR DISEASE CONTROL AND PREVENTION, 2016. *Lesson 1: Introduction to epidemiology* [viewed 4 January 2023]. Available from: www.cdc.gov/csels/dsepd/ss1978/Less on1/Section1.html

CENTERS FOR DISEASE CONTROL AND PREVENTION, 2022. *CDC's Building resilience against climate effects (BRACE) framework* [viewed 6 January 2023]. Available from:www.cdc.gov/climateandhealth/BRACE.htm

CHADWICK, E.,1842, *Sanitary condition of the labouring population of Great Britain: Report to Her Majesty's Principal Secretary of State for the Home Department from the Poor Law Commissioners, on an Inquiry into the sanitary condition of the labouring population of Great Britain*. London: Her Majesty's Stationery Office.

CHIOLERO, A. and D. BUCKERIDGE, 2020. Glossary for public health surveillance in the age of data. *Scientific journal of epidemiology and community health*, 74, 612–616. https://doi.org/10.1136/jech-2018-211654

DEPARTMENT OF HEALTH, 2009. *Stroke: Act F.A.S.T. awareness campaign* Available from: http://webarchive.nationalarchives.gov.uk/20130107105354/ www.dh.gov.uk/en/Publicationsandstatistics/Publications/PublicationsPolicyAndGuidance/DH_094239.

DUNN, J., R. RUNGE and N. SNYDER, 2018. Wearables and the medical revolution. *Personalized medicine*, 15(5), 429-448. https://doi.org/10.2217/pme-2018-0044

ENGELS, F., 1845/1993. *The condition of the working class in England. Oxford World's Classics*. Oxford: Oxford University Press

FACULTY OF PUBLIC HEALTH, 2016. *UK Faculty of Public Health strategy 2019–2025*. London: Faculty of Public Health.

FRY, D. and A. ZASK, 2017. Applying the Ottawa Charter to inform health promotion programme design. *Health promotion international*, 32(5), 901-912. https://doi.org/10.1093/heapro/daw022

HANLON, P. *et al.*, 2011. Making the case for a 'fifth wave' in public health. *Public health*, 125(1), 30–36. https://doi.org/10.1016/j.puhe.2010.09.004

HEALTH FOUNDATION, 2022. *Public Health Act 1875* [viewed 2 January 2023]. Available from: https://navigator.health.org.uk/theme/public-health-act-1875

HERNANDEZ, J. B. R. and P. Y. KIM, 2022. *Epidemiology morbidity and mortality*. Treasure Island, FL: StatPearls Publishing LLC.

INSTITUTE FOR APPRENTICESHIPS AND TECHNICAL EDUCATION, 2021. *Healthcare assistant practitioner* [viewed 7 January 2023]. Available from: www.instituteforapprenticeships.org/apprenticeship-standards/healthcare-assistant-practitioner-v1-0

JOHNSON, K. and M. L. BOVBJERG, 2020. *Foundations of epidemiology*. Oregon, USA: Oregon State University.

MARMOT, M., 2010. *Fair society, healthy Lives: The Marmot Review*. London: Institute of Health Equity.

MARMOT, M. *et al.*, 2020. *Health equity in England: The Marmot Review 10 years on*. London: Institute of Health Equity.

NATIONAL INSTITUTE FOR HEALTH AND CARE EXCELLENCE, 2023. *NICE and health inequalities* [viewed 4 January 2023]. Available from: www.nice.org.uk/about/what-we-do/nice-and-health-inequalities

NURSING AND MIDWIFERY COUNCIL (NMC), 2018. *The code: Professional standards of practice and behaviour for nurses, midwives and nursing associates* [viewed 25 September 2022]. Available from: www.nmc.org.uk/standards/code/

NUFFIELD COUNCIL ON BIOETHICS, 2007. *Public health: Ethical issues*. London: Nuffield Council on Bioethics.

PROCHASKA, J. O. and C. C. DICLEMENTE, 1984. *The transtheoretical approach: Crossing traditional boundaries of therapy*. Homewood, IL: Dow Jones Irwin.

RAINGRUBER, B., 2017. The history of health promotion. In B. Raingrubber, *Contemporary health promotion in nursing practice*, pp.23-47. Bolingbrook, IL: Jones and Bartlett Publishers, Inc.

SMITH, P. G., R. H. MORROW and D. A. ROSS, 2015. *Field trials of health interventions: A toolbox*. 3rd ed. Oxford: Oxford University Press.

SNOW, J., 1849. *On the mode of communication of cholera*. London: John Churchill.

TAM, C. and W. HAAS, 2016. *Outbreak investigations*. In: I. Abubakar, H. R. Stagg, T. Cohen, L. C. Rodrigues (eds.). *Infectious disease epidemiology*. Oxford: Oxford University Press.

THALER, R. H. and C. SUNSTEIN, 2008. *Nudge: Improving decisions about health, wealth, and happiness*. Yale: Yale University Press.

UK PARLIAMENT, 2022. *The 1848 Public Health Act* [viewed 4 January 2023]. Available from: www.parliament.uk/about/living-heritage/transformingsociety/towncountry/towns/tyne-and-wear-case-study/about-the-group/public-administration/the-1848-public-health-act/#:~:text=The%20Act%20established%20a%20Central,removal%20of%20nuisances%20and%20paving.

WINSLOW, C-E. A.,1920. The untilled fields of public health. *Science*, 51(1306), 23-33. https://doi.org/10.1126/science.51.1306.23

WORLD HEALTH ORGANIZATION, 2000. *World Health Organization world health report 2000*. Geneva: World Health Organization .

WORLD HEALTH ORGANIZATION, 2022. *Health promotion* [viewed 4 January 2023]. Geneva: World Health Organization. Available from: www.who.int/health-topics/health-promotion#tab=tab_1

13 Service improvement in health and social care

Lisa Arai

Box 13.1: Contents

- Introduction
- What does 'service improvement' mean?
- Why is service improvement necessary in health and social care?
- Completing your service improvement project
- Stage 1: Starting out: What is the opportunity or problem?
- Stage 2: Design and plan: What does the future look like?
- Stage 3: Implement, evaluate and disseminate
- General advice for students engaged in service improvement

Box 13.2: Learning outcomes

By the end of this chapter, you should be able to

- Define service improvement
- Discuss the drivers of service improvement
- Identify some of the methods, models and tools used in service improvement
- Demonstrate knowledge of the steps involved in completing your own, small-scale health and social care service improvement project.

Box 13.3: Keywords

- Service improvement
- Quality improvement
- Implementation
- Errors

DOI: 10.4324/9781003198338-17

- Waste
- Evaluation
- Lean
- Plan, do, study, act (PDSA)
- Nudge theory
- Stakeholders
- Gantt chart

Introduction

This chapter aims to examine service improvement in health and social care (H&SC). We will explore what the term 'service improvement' means and examine related terms such as 'quality improvement'. There are many tools and frameworks to guide would-be service improvers; some of these will be examined here. While many service improvement projects are large-scale, resource-intensive and long-running, the focus here is on the completion of brief, small-scale and low-cost (or no-cost) projects, the kinds of projects that students complete as part of a H&SC foundation degree, like the one we run at Solent University. This chapter refers to this programme, utilises insights from teaching on the service improvement module and refers to some of the projects Solent learners have completed over the years.

What does service improvement mean?

Defining service improvement

Activity 13.1: What is service improvement?

Jot down, in one or two sentences, what you think the term 'service improvement' means.

Service improvement is about making services less wasteful, more efficient and more responsive to the needs of staff, patients and service users. The term 'service improvement' tends to be used less frequently than 'quality improvement', which is described in a much-cited definition as: 'The combined efforts of everyone to make changes, leading to better patient outcomes (health), better system performance (care) and better professional development (learning) regardless of the theoretical concept or tool utilised' (Batalden and Davidoff 2007, p.2). More recently, Alderwick *et al.* (2017) referred to quality improvement as involving the: '... use of methods and tools to continuously improve quality of care and outcomes for patients'. Other related terms include 'quality enhancement' or 'service enhancement'. Lucas and Nacer (2015) refer to 'improving quality' and, in their discussion of the related field of 'improvement science', Moonesinghe and Peden (2017) write that this term can be used interchangeably with quality improvement but argue that these are separate disciplines.

Service improvement in health and social care

As Craig (2018) observes, the idea of improving quality in H&SC is not a contemporary idea, noting that the first clinical audits were carried out in the 1900s. While not a new discipline, the history of healthcare quality before 1960 has been described as a: '… fragmented collection of unrelated events rather than a streamlined organized effort' (Sheingold and Hahn 2014, p.18). Sheingold and Hahn (2014) argue that this history is now taken-for-granted because it's so 'embedded' in everyday healthcare practice and quality improvement activities. These authors point to Florence Nightingale (among others) as a pioneer of quality improvement. She helped reduce cholera- and diarrhoea-associated mortality rates among soldiers fighting in the Crimean War, from 43% to 2% through the introduction of comparatively simple measures (reduction of overcrowding, better ventilation and disinfection of latrines).

As several commentators have noted, many contemporary service and quality improvement methods and approaches were originally developed in industry and have been adapted for H&SC settings (Craig 2018; Jones, Kwong and Warburton 2021). However, Craig expresses concern about the use of 'business-like' approaches to service improvement, arguing these have: '… failed to account for the complexity of health care and have been labelled by staff as management fads…' (p.893).

Panel 13.1: Lean thinking

Lean thinking was developed from the Toyota Production System and is widely used in many areas, especially the National Health Service. It identifies ways to reduce waste and provide better outcomes without additional resources.

Read more about Lean thinking in the National Health Service in the National Health Service Institute for Innovation and Improvement (2007) at: www.england. nhs.uk/improvement-hub/wp-content/uploads/sites/44/2017/11/Going-Lean-in-the-NHS.pdf

---

As you can see from this brief discussion, even defining service improvement and understanding its relationship to other, related, activities and processes is not straightforward. The term 'service improvement' is used here because it is one of the more straightforward and widely understood terms, and this chapter draws on a module taught at Solent University with that title, but please be aware of the usage of the other terms.

Activity 13.2: Research, audit and service improvement

While service improvement is not the same as a research project or an audit, service improvement projects usually include the completion of audits, and learners engaged in service improvement typically use research methods to collect and analyse data.

Read: an overview of the differences between these and other activities in the National Patient Safety Agency (2010) guide at: www.uhbristol.nhs.uk/media/1572 809/defining_research_leaflet_1_.pdf

Service improvement in policy and practice

Contemporary H&SC practitioners are likely to be very aware of the importance of service improvement in their workplaces; service or quality improvement is often an essential activity in a practitioner's role. Service improvement has also been referred to in various policy documents including the Berwick Report (National Advisory Group on the Safety of Patients in England 2013), the Francis Report (2013) and the National Health Service (NHS) Long-Term Plan (NHS 2019). The authors of the latter write that:

> Delivering the Long-Term Plan will rely on local healthcare systems having the capability to implement change effectively. Systematic methods of quality improvement (QI) provide an evidence-based approach for improving every aspect of how the NHS operates. Through developing their improvement capabilities, including QI skills and data analytics, systems will move further and faster to adopt new innovations and service models and implement best practices that can improve quality and efficiency and reduce unwarranted variations in performance (NHS 2019, p.111).

The Willis review (2015) expressed a desire for newly qualified nurses to be able to lead service improvement projects, thus improving the quality of care given to patients.

To do this, the review authors said: '...registered nurses will need the knowledge and analytical skills to make informed decisions and contribute effectively to new innovations, taking a more proactive role in service improvement change and change management' (p.26). Similarly, Smith, Pearson and Adams (2014) maintain that service improvement must be an integral part of all nurses' approach to caregiving: 'The preparation of undergraduate nursing students must keep abreast of current developments in healthcare if the students are going to function effectively in their clinical posts upon qualification' (p.624). These authors note that, although service improvement projects are an important part of the clinical culture of the NHS in England, it took longer for them to be regarded as an integral part of undergraduate pre-registration healthcare programmes.

Why is service improvement necessary in health and social care?

Thus far, we have defined service improvement, briefly considered its history and looked at the policy context. Why, though, is service improvement necessary? What are the pressures on contemporary healthcare systems that make service improvement so important? As Lucas and Nacer (2015) observe, H&SC professionals' education and training do not properly equip them for today's or tomorrow's 'ever-changing healthcare settings' (p.6). What can we say about the nature of these healthcare settings? In what ways are they 'ever-changing'?

Drivers of service improvement

In this section, we will examine some of the drivers for service improvement in H&SC in the United Kingdom (UK; although it's important to be aware that many other countries' healthcare systems—especially those in higher-income countries—are affected by the same pressures). What are the drivers for service improvement?

Demographic factors

The first factor is demographic and is primarily related to increases in population size and the number of older people in the population. When the NHS was created in 1946 (it started operating in 1948), the UK was a very different country than the one it is today. For one, life expectancy was much lower. In 1948, it was approximately 66 years for men and 70 years for women. Nearly 70 years later, men can expect to live to nearly 80 years and women to 83 years (Nuffield Trust 2018). Older patients make greater demands of services, and their needs are more complex. Patients with multiple morbidities—individuals who have two or more chronic or long-term conditions occurring simultaneously (McGeorge 2018; National Institute for Health and Care Excellence 2016) —present special challenges. Two-thirds of people aged 65 years and over have multiple morbidities (National Institute for Health and Care Excellence 2016). One of the main issues for this population group include polypharmacy ('… the concurrent use of multiple medications by one individual'; King's Fund 2013, p.9). Multiple appointments and unplanned care are other salient care issues (National Institute for Health and Care Excellence 2016).

Costs

The cost of the NHS has continued to increase over many decades, ever since it began operating in July 1948. Harker (2019) notes that, in the first full year of its operation, the Government spent nearly £11.4 billion in today's prices on health; by 2018/2019, the figure was more than ten times that, at £152.9 billion. Harker writes that: '…between 2000/2001 and 2004/2005, the average annual spending growth was 8.7%, which is higher than that at any other time in the history of the NHS' (p.3).

Much of this expenditure is because of staff costs; in 2019/2020, NHS staff cost was around £56 billion, which is 46.6% of the NHS budget (King's Fund 2022). Increased expenditure is also associated with advances in medical treatment. The most expensive medical treatments (in vitro fertilisation, organ transplantation, foetal ultrasound, use of pacemakers, etc.) were not available when the NHS was created.

Errors, inefficiency and waste

According to some commentators, the NHS is wasteful and inefficient. Responding to the Carter review (2016) on performance in English NHS acute hospitals and which identified significant unwarranted variation between settings, the Tax Payers' Alliance (TPA) wrote that:

> …the TPA views the publication of the Carter Review as a reinforcement of what we have known for some time: there is waste in the system… the first step in safeguarding the NHS finances would be to cut out the waste so that tax payers' money can be focused on patient care (Tax Payers' Alliance 2016).

More recently, a TPA report (Cook 2022) highlighted differences across the NHS in England in estate costs (cost associated with running and maintaining buildings) and, in the Prime Minister's Spring Statement, Rishi Sunak announced efforts to tackle waste and inefficiency across the public sector including the NHS (Chancellor of the Exchequer 2022).

Panel 13.2: Medication errors

Elliott *et al.* (2018) undertook a rapid evidence synthesis and economic analysis of the prevalence and burden of medication error. Their report found that:

- Over 237 million medication errors occur during the medication process in England in 1 year. Most (72.1%), however, of these were minor, with little or no potential for clinical harm
- Nearly 66 million potentially clinically significant errors occurred, most of which (71%) occurred in primary care
- Primary care prescribing accounted for nearly 34% of all potentially clinically significant errors
- The estimated burden of errors was £98.5 million per annum, causing 712 deaths and contributing to 1,708 deaths.

Read the review at: https://drive.google.com/file/d/1tHw-R4Q9BtXNepHny CM8DzMWjsySavp1/view?usp=sharing

---

Patient and service user expectations

Duffy (2018) notes that, while a significant number of people think the standard of care offered by the NHS is poor, the British public is committed to its continuation:

> Eight in ten say the NHS is crucial to British society and we must do everything to maintain it in its current form. Around nine in ten are committed to ensuring the NHS is free at the point of access and provides a comprehensive service to everyone.

Duffy maintains that the public's high expectations of the NHS are related, in part, to their experiences of 'sophisticated, speedy and personalised services in the private sector'. The question is: will these high expectations of the NHS continue in the face of the many challenges it faces and, moreover, can they be met? These questions were especially salient during the post-COVID-19 period. The COVID-19-related care backlog means routine operations, for example, are likely to be affected for years (King's Fund 2022).

These diverse factors—demographic, economic, behavioural and attitudinal—are the main drivers of service improvement and form the backdrop to contemporary service improvement initiatives. Together, they have contributed to a sense of H&SC services as being under immense strain and are only likely to intensify in the coming years. H&SC workers have little power to bring about the kind of deep change needed for the NHS to function optimally, but they can, in small but significant and meaningful ways, play a role in making services more efficient and attuned to the needs of patients.

Completing your service improvement project

If you complete a service improvement module as part of your educational or training programme, you will design, implement and evaluate a small-scale project in your own workplace. Because of time and resource constraints, these projects must necessarily be small-scale and have low or no cost attached to them. They must also not be ethically problematic (see chapters 3 and 11). Moreover, the service improvement project must be pragmatic, feasible and clinically important or relevant.

Solent University's Service Improvement Project module

All Solent University students are in practice when they commence study on the foundation degree in H&SC programme and are either trainee nursing associates or healthcare assistant practitioners. Towards the end of level 5 (second year), they must design, implement and evaluate a small-scale service improvement project as part of their training. As noted above, this must be at low or no cost, and managers must approve the project. The projects are written up in the form of posters and students are invited to a viva, a defence of their work, where they are asked questions of their project and invited to speak about the project more generally. We encourage the students to think of the project rather than the poster. The poster is the reporting of the project and, regardless of how well designed or colourful the poster is, if the project isn't coherent, the poster is not likely to be.

Because our practitioner students design, implement and evaluate these projects in real-world settings, the module can be challenging to complete. Our H&SC learners work in busy clinical settings, are nearly always practising under time and other constraints and can sometimes experience unexpected changes in the workplace (a new job role, a change of manager).

What kinds of projects have our students developed? You can see examples of the types of projects completed by students in Panel 13.3.

Panel 13.3: Examples of service improvement projects by Solent University health and social care students

Over the many years Solent University's health and social care students have been undertaking service improvement projects, we've seen a diverse array of projects focused on reducing waste, increasing efficiency and helping teams work more efficiently. Here's a selection of the type of projects learners have completed:

- Laminated guidance on calculating the National Early Warning Score (NEWS2) (a system standardising assessment of, and response to, acute illness; Royal College of Physicians 2017)
- Redesign of an existing checklist to ensure staff complete blood pressure tests on patients on admittance to a general adult ward
- Patient information notice board in a paediatric ward advising patients of clinic opening times, location of amenities such as toilets and the canteen and how to contact staff to discuss concerns
- Creation of a data collection tool to be used by staff when recording observations of high-risk patients in an acute mental health setting
- Staff training to raise awareness of the nursing associate role in a children's palliative care setting
- Change to clinic times to reduce non-attendance in a maternity care setting
- Brief lunchtime training to help staff understand the nutritional needs of patients with type 2 diabetes

- Colourful and engaging poster displayed prominently above sinks in accident and emergency to encourage effective handwashing among staff
- Brightly coloured, removable stickers placed on equipment reminding staff to clean it between patients
- Campaign (poster, brief training) to remind maternity staff to remove jewellery below the elbow before clinical work commences
- A laminated poster placed in an operating theatre reminding surgeons and other clinical staff of the correct way to wear protective eyewear.

How do students complete these projects? What approaches and tools do students utilise? We will discuss these now.

Service improvement frameworks and tools

Stages in the service improvement process

Solent University students use a worksheet containing a modified version of NHS England's six-stage quality and service improvement project management approach (NHS England 2022) when they are designing their projects. The version our students use has the following stages:

- Stage 1: Starting out: What is the opportunity or problem?
- Stage 2: Design and plan: What does the future look like?
- Stage 3: Implement, evaluate and disseminate

Students complete the worksheet on a week-by-week basis while the module is in progress. The worksheet has proven to be an invaluable tool in supporting students through the service improvement design process. We will now look at each of the three stages below and highlight selected tools and frameworks that can be used at each stage.

Stage 1: Starting out: What is the opportunity or problem?

At the first stage of the process, students are asked to identify the nature of the problem and to consider why it happens. The specific areas that students examine are:

- The project setting: This should be briefly described in the poster. Students are reminded not to assume that the viewers of the poster will understand the type of clinical setting they work in or what happens in the work setting. A brief description of the clinical setting for the improvement project helps contextualise it and 'sets the scene' for what follows. Students can also briefly refer to any recent significant changes that might affect their own improvement projects ('The service was re-organised a year ago to meet increased demand and, since then, the number of staff has increased')
- Evidence-based rationale for the project: all service improvement projects should have a strong rationale; there must be a reason why the change is needed. Students should demonstrate the importance of, and reason for, the service improvement in their posters and in the viva. Recent relevant research and other information should be

drawn on to support the rationale and to ensure the project is evidence-based. In addition, our students complete an audit before the module commences so that they can measure what happens in practice before they implement change. They are encouraged to draw on this at this stage of the process to strengthen the rationale.

Panel 13.4: What is an audit?

An audit is a: '...way to find out if healthcare is being provided in line with standards and lets care providers and patients know where their service is doing well, and where there could be improvements' (NHS England 2019).

- Aim of the project: the aim should be clear by reading the poster title. Our students are advised that only one (well developed and refined) aim is needed; vague, 'woolly' aims mean a vague, 'woolly' project. The rationale (if well made) helps 'make space' for the project aim. For example: 'The audit completed before the project commenced showed that 15% of in-patients with type 2 diabetes (T2DM) had not eaten properly in the 6- hour period being monitored. This can have adverse health and other impacts in this group. Therefore, the aim of this project is to develop a paper-based tool to remind staff to check on the eating habits of in-patients with T2DM'.

Panel 13.5: Writing aims and titles

Aims and titles are different—an aim is a statement about what you hope to achieve, a title is the name of a project—but each contain the same elements, or it can be confusing for people viewing posters or other outputs of a service improvement project.

For example, if David's project aim is: 'To improve handwashing among staff in a general adult ward through implementation of a service improvement project', the title can be written as: 'Improving handwashing practices among staff in a general adult ward: Findings from a service improvement project'.

If Hassan's project aim is: 'To improve collection of observational data in an adult intensive care unit', the title can be written as: 'A project to improve collection of observational data in an adult intensive care unit'.

Go to: www.england.nhs.uk/wp-content/uploads/2021/03/qsir-developing-your-aims-statement.pdf

---

- Linkage of the project to the student's organisation's strategic goals: As stated earlier, Solent University students are supported by their managers and workplace colleagues in planning their service improvement projects. In fact, it would be impossible to implement their projects without the support of colleagues so it's imperative that students recognise this in their projects. One way to do this is to draw on their organisations' strategic goals. These are developed to help guide the direction of the organisation and are often linked to national policy. Strategic goals are often quite general in nature ('Provide compassionate, patient-centred care'), so it's not usually difficult to align projects with strategic goals and can be found on the organisation's website.

Activity 13.3: Find your organisation's strategic goals

Go to the website of your Trust or other health and social care organisation. If you are not working in a health and social care setting, then look at the website of your local Trust. Can you find the organisation's strategic goals? What do these say? See NHS England and NHS Improvement (2021a).

- Benefit to others as a result of the proposed change: Learners should specify how others will benefit from the proposed change. 'Others' here includes patients, service users or staff. While Solent University's students can consider specific patient health outcomes (better nutrition, better management of a condition like asthma) they are advised that this is not a health promotion project so they should focus on the service itself.

Panel 13.6: Understanding why problems arise

One way to understand why and how problems arise is to use the fishbone tool. This aids in understanding the cause and effect. You can read more about this tool at NHS England and NHS Improvement's (2021b) guide at: www.england.nhs.uk/wp-content/uploads/2021/12/qsir-cause-and-effect-fishbone.pdf

---

Stage 2: Design and plan: What does the future look like?

Having completed stage 1 of the worksheet, students then move into the design phase of the process where students consider:

- The type of service improvement change and the steps involved in the change: Even with the smallest service improvement project, it's important to be clear about the method to bring about change. This needs to make sense in light of the audit findings and the nature of the problem identified. If, for example, the audit findings show a lack of awareness among staff of the need to complete an activity, then a training initiative might be introduced to raise awareness. If the audit results demonstrate that staff are struggling to complete an existing checklist because it's confusing or too long, then the change might be the redesign of the checklist.
- Students should also specify the steps involved in the proposed change. For example, one student, Lizzie, noticed that residents with type 2 diabetes (T2DM) in the care home where she worked were accidentally being given the same meals as residents without

T2DM even though their nutritional needs were different. She audited occasions when T2DM patients received the wrong meals, collected data from staff about why this happened and decided that a sticker placed prominently on the front of patient notes, accompanied by a 5-minute awareness raising session, would help to remind busy staff during mealtime about which of the residents had T2DM. Even this kind of simple change needed to be designed, so Lizzie had to explain why and how the sticker was developed (drawing on the research evidence) and the content of the 5-minute session.

Panel 13.7: The role of theory in service improvement

In many service improvement projects, the planned change will often involve a degree of behavioural change (Davidoff *et al.*, 2015). For example: In a project to encourage disposal of waste in the correct bin in a hospital, the student plans to place a coloured arrow above each bin to remind staff about which bin they should use. The student hopes that seeing the arrow will translate into behavioural change.

One theory that Solent University students are taught is 'Nudge'. Nudge was developed by two United Stated–based behavioural economists (Thaler and Sunstein 2008) and argues that people can be encouraged to make better (or healthier) choices through often small modifications to the environment and provision of incentives.

Activity 13.4: Plan, do, study, act (PDSA)

Plan, do, study, act cycles are widely used in quality and service improvement projects. The use of this cycle facilitates testing out of proposed changes on a smaller scale before full implementation. PDSA stands for:

- Plan the change to be implemented
- Do carry out the change
- Study–collect data before and after the change to assess the impact of the change
- Act–plan the next change cycle or full implementation.

Go to NHS England and NHS Improvement's (2022a) guidance on this cycle at: www.england.nhs.uk/wp-content/uploads/2022/01/qsir-pdsa-cycles-model-for-improvement.pdf
Read more about this tool. Can you see how you can use several PDSA cycles in the lifetime of one project?

- The project stakeholders: stakeholders are '… anyone who has an interest in a project and can influence its success or failure …' as described by Silver *et al.* (2016, p.893). They also say that it's important to identify stakeholders who can affect the project at an early stage when: '… these relationships can be managed' and that stakeholders can include supporters and 'resistors of change' (Silver *et al.* 2016, p.893). 'Resistors of change' are people who (as the term implies) resist change, usually because they have 'done things' the same way for many years and may see change as threatening.

Activity 13.5: Stakeholder analysis

Go to NHS England and NHS Improvement's (2022b) stakeholder analysis at: www/ england.nhs.uk/wp-content/uploads/2022/02/qsir-stakeholder-analysis.pdf
   Read about the five stages of stakeholder analysis. Can you think of any stakeholders for your service improvement project? This can be an actual project or a hypothetical one.

- The stages in the project: Students are advised to create a Gantt chart showing each stage of the project, from inception to dissemination.

Stage 3: Implement, evaluate and disseminate

In the final stage of the three-part process, students examine:

- Who will be involved in implementation of the change: While individuals should not be named, specific roles ('ward sister' 'healthcare assistants') can be referred to
- Barriers and levers to implementation: Students are asked to think about factors that might hinder the project. The Health Foundation (de Silva 2015) observes that barriers can often be about the change itself (a re-designed data collection form might be too complicated to use, for example) or maybe the proposed change is not compatible with existing systems (this is more likely to happen with technology-based changes) or is perceived to be no better than alternatives. Other common barriers to implementation include not allocating enough time or resources to the project or practical barriers (such as space constraints). Levers to implementation are factors facilitating the project, the chief of which is the support of managers and colleagues (NHS England and NHS Improvement 2022c)
- Evaluation of the effects of the change: Students are asked to re-audit their projects post-implementation. Usually, they will use the same methods they used with the first audit. Some students decide to collect additional data on, for example, colleagues' views of the change. This kind of information is especially useful if the project didn't lead to the expected outcomes
- Dissemination of findings: As noted above, Solent University students discuss their project in the context of a viva attended by staff and colleagues, including managers. The latter are often keen to see the students' work disseminated more widely, beyond the student's primary place of work. Therefore, students are asked to devise a dissemination strategy. The strategy is hypothetical, of course, as dissemination takes place after the module has finished. Feedback from former students suggests that many of these dissemination activities do, in fact, take place and many service improvement projects are extended either within the original service setting or rolled out to other

settings. Some of our students become service improvement 'champions' and have presented their findings at conferences and other events.

Activity 13.6: Creating a dissemination strategy

Create a dissemination strategy for an actual or hypothetical service improvement project. Use the template shown below to do this (the first row has already been completed).

Type of dissemination activity	Audience	Aim	Content	Materials	Location and date
Seminar	Ward staff	To report selected project findings	Background to project, interim findings	Slides, re-designed leaflet	Ward, June

---

General advice for students engaged in service improvement

At Solent University, we've found that using the three stages of the service improvement approach described above, and by signposting our students to the many quality and service improvement and frameworks tools (especially those at NHS England at: www.england.nhs.uk/sustainableimprovement/qsir-programme/qsir-tools/) helps learner think about *all* the steps involved in service improvement. These tools and approaches also help give the module focus for could be, otherwise, a challenging experience.

What other (more general) tips can be helpful for service improvers (especially those in practice). These include:

- Remember that small scale does not mean small impact: service improvement projects must have no cost attached, they must not cause inconvenience to staff or patients and they have to be completed within a short span of time, so they are necessarily small scale, but this does not mean they have limited impact. Many students tell us that their projects have been positively received and that they plan to develop their projects further and roll them out to a wider range of clinical settings
- Ask colleagues for help: our students are on placement for part of the time they are working on their projects. This has implications for data collection (for the audit and re-audit). We advise students to ask colleagues to collect data on their behalf if they cannot
- Mistakes are good: this especially holds true when a service improvement change does not have its hoped-for impact. This may be because for some of the reasons discussed above (limitations in design, problems with fault in implementation, etc.). However, it's important to acknowledge the project's limitations and to consider how the project might be modified and re-implemented (NHS England and NHS Improvement 2021c)

- Be prepared to experience resistance or challenges: it can be difficult for H&SC students to challenge practice (or to be seen to be challenging practice). Identifying personal styles is the key to understanding others and to address concerns they may have with the project (NHS England and NHS Improvement 2022c).

Summary

This chapter defined service improvement, briefly considered its history and the policy context and examined some of the drivers of service improvement. Students working to change an aspect of their clinical setting may not be able to cause large-scale profound changes, especially against a backdrop of pressures on the service related to demands, resourcing and unexpected events such as COVID-19, but they can make small changes to their practice or clinical service to make it more efficient or less wasteful. We discussed selected service improvement tools and frameworks here, drawing on a three-stage framework that H&SC students use on the service improvement module at Solent University.

Box 13.4: Key learning points

- Service improvement is about making services less wasteful, more efficient and more responsive to the needs of people working in or using the services
- Many contemporary service improvement methods and approaches were originally developed in industry and have been adapted for care settings
- There are several drivers of service improvement—demographic, economic, behavioural and attitudinal. These drivers form the backdrop to contemporary service improvement initiatives and, together, have contributed to a sense of services as being under strain
- Solent University students use a modified worksheet to complete their projects, which has three stages: What is the opportunity or problem; what does the future look like and implement, evaluate and disseminate.

References

ALDERWICK, H. *et al.*, 2017. *Making the case for quality improvement: Lessons for NHS boards and leaders* [viewed 2 January 2022]. Available from: www.kingsfund.org.uk/publications/making-case-quality-improvement

BATALDEN, P. B. and F. DAVIDOFF, 2007. What is 'quality improvement' and how can it transform healthcare? *Quality and safety in health care*, 16(1), 2-3. https://doi.org/10.1136/qshc.2006.022046

CARTER, L., 2016. *Operational productivity and performance in English NHS acute hospitals: Unwarranted variations.* London: Crown copyright.

CHANCELLOR OF THE EXCHEQUER, 2022. *Spring statement.* CP 653. London: Crown Copyright.

COOK, S., 2022. *An analysis of hospital estates spending in the English NHS.* London: TPA.

CRAIG, L., 2018. Service improvement in health care: A literature review. *British journal of nursing*, 27(15), 893-896. https://doi.org/10.12968/bjon.2018.27.15.893

DAVIDOFF, F. *et al.*, 2015. Demystifying theory and its use in improvement. *BMJ quality and safety*, 24(3), 228-238. https://doi.org/10.1136/bmjqs-2014-003627

de Silva, D., 2015. *What's getting in the way? Barriers to improvement in the NHS.* London: Health Foundation.

DUFFY, B., 2018. *Public expectations of the NHS* [King's Fund blog] [viewed 25 September 2022]. Available from: www.kingsfund.org.uk/blog/2018/02/public-expectations-nhs

ELLIOTT, J. *et al.*, 2018. *Prevalence and economic burden of medication errors in the NHS in England. Rapid evidence synthesis and economic analysis of the prevalence and burden of medication error in the UK.* Universities of Sheffield and York: Policy Research Unit in Economic Evaluation of Health and Care Interventions.

FRANCIS, R., 2013. *Report of the Mid Staffordshire NHS Foundation Trust Public Inquiry. Volume 1: Analysis of evidence and lessons learned (part 1)* [viewed 31 December 2022]. Available from: https://assets.publishing.service.gov.uk/government/uploads/system/uploads/attachment_data/file/279115/0898_i.pdf

HARKER, R., 2019. *NHS funding and expenditure.* Briefing paper, CBP0724. London: House of Commons Library.

JONES, B., E. KWONG and W. WARBURTON, 2021. *Quality improvement made simple: What everyone should know about health care quality improvement.* London: The Health Foundation.

KING'S FUND, 2022. *Key facts and figures about the NHS* [viewed 2 January 2023]. Available from: www.kingsfund.org.uk/audio-video/key-facts-figures-nhs

LUCAS, B. and H. NACER, 2015. *The habits of an improver: Thinking about learning for improvement in health care.* London: Health Foundation.

MCGEORGE, S., 2018. *Morbidity–comorbidity and multimorbidity. What do they mean?* [viewed 2 January 2023]. Available from: www.bgs.org.uk/resources/morbidity-comorbidity-and-multimorbidity-what-do-they-mean

MOONESINGHE, S. R. and C. J. PEDEN, 2017. Theory and context: Putting the science into improvement. *British journal of anaesthesia,* 118(4), 482-484. https://doi.org/10.1093/bja/aew469

NATIONAL ADVISORY GROUP ON THE SAFETY OF PATIENTS IN ENGLAND (BERWICK REPORT), 2013. *Improving the safety of patients in England.* London: Crown Copyright.

NATIONAL INSTITUTE FOR HEALTH AND CARE EXCELLENCE, 2016. *Multimorbidity: Clinical assessment and management: Multimorbidity: assessment, prioritisation and management of care for people with commonly occurring multimorbidity* (NICE guideline NG56). London: National Institute for Health and Care Excellence.

NATIONAL PATIENT SAFETY AGENCY, 2010. *Defining research* [viewed 2 January 2023]. Available from: www.uhbristol.nhs.uk/media/1572809/defining_research_leaflet_1_.pdf

NHS, 2019. *The NHS Long Term Plan.* London: HMSO.

NHS ENGLAND, 2019. *Clinical audit* [viewed 2 January 2023]. Available from: www.england.nhs.uk/clinaudit/

NHS ENGLAND, 2022. *Quality, service improvement and redesign (QSIR) tools by stage of project* [viewed 2 January 2023]. Available from: www.england.nhs.uk/sustainableimprovement/qsir-programme/qsir-tools/tools-by-stage-of-project/

NHS ENGLAND AND NHS IMPROVEMENT, 2021a. *Aligning improvement with strategic goals* [viewed 2 January 2023]. Available from: www.england.nhs.uk/wp-content/uploads/2021/03/qsir-aligning-improvement-strategic-goals.pdf

NHS ENGLAND AND NHS IMPROVEMENT, 2021b. *Cause and effect (fishbone)* [viewed 2 January 2023]. Available from: www.england.nhs.uk/wp-content/uploads/2021/12/qsir-cause-and-effect-fishbone.pdf

NHS ENGLAND AND NHS IMPROVEMENT, 2021c. *Reviving a stalled effort* [viewed 2 January 2023]. Available from: www.england.nhs.uk/wp-content/uploads/2021/03/qsir-reviving-stalled-effort.pdf

NHS ENGLAND AND NHS IMPROVEMENT, 2022a. *Plan, do, study, act (PDSA) cycles and the model for improvement* [viewed 2 January 2023]. Available from: www.england.nhs.uk/wp-content/uploads/2022/01/qsir-pdsa-cycles-model-for-improvement.pdf

NHS ENGLAND AND NHS IMPROVEMENT, 2022b. *Stakeholder analysis* [viewed 2 January 2023]. Available from: www.england.nhs.uk/wp-content/uploads/2022/02/qsir-stakeholder-analysis.pdf

NHS ENGLAND AND NHS IMPROVEMENT, 2022c. *How to understand differences between individuals* [viewed 2 January 2023]. Available from: www.england.nhs.uk/wp-content/uploads/2022/01/qsir-understand-differences-between-individuals.pdf

NHS INSTITUTE FOR INNOVATION AND IMPROVEMENT, 2007. *Going lean in the NHS* [viewed 2 January 2023]. Available from: www.england.nhs.uk/improvement-hub/wp-content/uploads/sites/44/2017/11/Going-Lean-in-the-NHS.pdf

NUFFIELD TRUST, 2018. *Facts and figures on the NHS at 70*. London: Nuffield Trust.

ROYAL COLLEGE OF PHYSICIANS, 2017. *National Early Warning Score (NEWS) 2 Standardising the assessment of acute-illness severity in the NHS* [viewed 2 January 2023]. Available from: www.rcplondon.ac.uk/file/8504/download

SHEINGOLD, B. H. and J. A. HAHN, 2014. The history of healthcare quality: The first 100 years 1860–1960. *International journal of Africa nursing sciences*, 1, 18-22. https://doi.org/10.1016/j.ijans.2014.05.002

SILVER, S. A. et al., 2016. How to begin a quality improvement project. *Clinical journal of the American society of nephrology*, 11(5), 893-900. https://doi.org/10.2215/CJN.11491015

SMITH, J., L. PEARSON and J. ADAMS, 2014. Incorporating a service improvement project into an undergraduate nursing programme: A pilot study. *International journal of nursing practice*, 20(6), 623-628. https://doi.org/10.1111/ijn.12217

TAX PAYERS' ALLIANCE (TPA), 2016. *Further proof of NHS waste* [viewed 2 January 2022]. Available from: www.taxpayersalliance.com/there_is_waste_in_the_system

THALER, R. H. and C. SUNSTEIN, 2008. *Nudge: Improving decisions about health, wealth, and happiness*. Yale: Yale University Press.

WILLIS, L., 2015. *Raising the bar: Shape of caring: A review of the future education and training of registered nurses and care assistants*. London: Health Education England/Nursing and Midwifery Council.

Index

Milton Keynes UK
Ingram Content Group UK Ltd.
UKHW051537141024
449569UK00028B/1507